I Left My Prostate in San Francisco—Where's Yours?

I Left My Prostate in San Francisco—

Where's Yours?

Coping with the Emotional,
Relational, Sexual, and Spiritual
Aspects of Prostate Cancer

Rick Redner and Brenda Redner

WestBow
PRESS
A DIVISION OF THOMAS NELSON

WestBow Press books may be ordered through
booksellers or by contacting:

WestBow Press
A Division of Thomas Nelson
1663 Liberty Drive
Bloomington, IN 47403
www.westbowpress.com
1-(866) 928-1240

NKJV – New King James Version
Scripture taken from the New King James Version.
Copyright 1979, 1980, 1982 by Thomas Nelson,
inc. Used by permission. All rights reserved.

Library of Congress Control Number: 2012923605

ISBN: 978-1-4497-7961-0 (sc)
ISBN: 978-1-4497-7960-3 (e)
ISBN: 978-1-4497-7962-7 (hc)

Printed in the United States of America

WestBow Press rev. date: 02/08/2013

Contents

Acknowledgments

I'd like to thank my wife, who encouraged me when I was discouraged, who loved me when I felt unlovable, who never doubted me, even when I doubted myself, who was persistent when I was ready to quit, and who believed we'd get through when I thought we were stuck. Thank you for being a godly helper. Thank you for staying by my side in sickness and in health.

I love you.

I'm also grateful to my family—Ryan, Andy, Chris, Kate, and Bre—for their support, understanding, kindness, and prayers. In your own way, each of you played an important role in helping me get out of the house at a time when my greatest desire was to stay home and withdraw from the world.

To all our friends and family who took the time to pray for us, visit, or keep in touch by phone, with cards, and through e-mails—all of you have my gratitude for the support and encouragement you gave us when our burden became too heavy for us to carry alone.

I'd also like to thank every health-care professional, from the urologists and surgeons to those doing research and those directly involved in patient care, such as the nurses and orderlies. May God bless you and everyone involved in treatment and prevention of prostate cancer.

Introduction

With the advent of yearly PSA testing and regular digital exams, we live in an era where men are frequently diagnosed with the early stages of prostate cancer. From a treatment perspective, this is great news. From an emotional standpoint, it's devastating. For men, this means, without warning or symptoms, you can move from being healthy one day to discovering you have a potentially life-threatening disease the next. This rapid, unexpected, and unwanted transition is emotionally overwhelming and hard to grasp.

I'm personally familiar with the anxiety or fear you feel if you or someone you love hears four words that will shatter his world: "You have prostate cancer."

I vividly remember the Sunday I received the phone call from my urologist. He told me my biopsy confirmed I had prostate cancer. Instantly, my world was turned upside down. It was the worst day of my life. The diagnosis of cancer brought images of pain, suffering, and death. I had no idea how aggressive my cancer was or whether it had spread to other parts of my body. I was terrified.

Questions popped into my mind, and I filled in the blanks. Here's how that went:

- *How long do I have left to live?* "Not long. This disease will kill me within a year."

- *Will I live long enough to see my daughter married?* "No, I won't live long enough to walk her down the aisle."

- *Will I be able to continue working?* "Not for long. I'd better put my business up for sale as quickly as possible. I might not live long enough to sell it."
- *Will the cost of treatment ruin us financially?* "Yes it will."
- *Will I suffer?* "Oh yeah."

I brought to my mind every ugly picture of cancer—suffering, pain, and dying—because I *knew* that was my future.

I pictured the cancer cells in my prostate as little "Pac-Men" with extremely sharp teeth working twenty-four/seven with one goal: to work their way through my prostate and kill me as quickly as possible. I wondered what dying from prostate cancer would be like. Sadly, most men keep their internal dialogue a secret. As men we feel a need to protect those we love. My definition of manhood kept me from sharing my thoughts with the very people who could have comforted me and shared my pain. My misguided definition of manhood led me to face my darkest fears alone.

I also lost the opportunity to correct my misperceptions. For example, it was weeks before I learned that cancer cells in my prostate were not like sharp-teethed Pac-Men. They were more like turtles. Since I lacked accurate information and knowledge, I wrongly assumed every minute that went by without treatment decreased my odds of survival. Therefore, I expected my urologist to refer me to the medical team that would treat my prostate cancer. That's not what happened. Instead he asked me how I wanted to treat my prostate cancer.

This made no sense to me. When my appendix became inflamed, or when I was diagnosed with a hernia, my doctor didn't ask me what type of treatment I wanted. He sent me to a surgeon. That's not true with prostate cancer. The decision is yours. I had a lot to learn, and I wanted to learn it fast so I could begin some form of treatment.

At a time when your emotions are out of control and you are facing your worst fears about cancer and/or dying, you have to make one of the most important decisions of your life, which is how to treat your prostate cancer. If you are like me, this is an overwhelming task. I had no idea where to begin. I only knew this much: I had to make an important, life-altering decision about a disease I knew absolutely nothing about.

Where do you begin? If you are Internet savvy, you'll probably use your favorite search engine and type in "treatment options for prostate cancer." When I did this, I discovered I had more than three million hits to my query. Upon further examination, many of these sites were promoting a specific treatment option. I wanted an objective analysis. There are thousands of excellent sites. I'll suggest just one—not because it's the best but because you need to start somewhere: http://www.cancer.gov/cancertopics/treatment/prostate/understanding-prostate-cancer-treatment/page1.

I went to the public library and took home more than a dozen books about prostate cancer. The best book I found was Dr. Patrick Walsh's *Guide to Surviving Prostate Cancer* (second edition). I highly recommend you purchase this book.

I've learned that the diagnosis of prostate cancer affects more than your physical health. Whichever treatment option you choose, you will also experience cancer's impact on the following areas of your life:

➤ **Your emotional life**: It can impact how you feel about yourself and your world.

➤ **Your psychological life**: It can affect how you think about yourself and your world.

➤ **Your relational life**: Every important relationship can be disrupted, such as your marriage and relationships with extended family members and friends.

- **Your spiritual life:** You may grow closer to or further away from God.

- **Your sexual life:** Surgery will result in temporary and permanent changes with regard to your sexuality and abilities.

Few books address all of these issues. My wife and I address all of them with three different perspectives. The first perspective comes from our personal experiences with prostate cancer. The second perspective comes from our professional training. The third perspective comes from our faith and biblically based worldview.

We believe men will do better and marriages will grow stronger when there is an accurate understanding of the physical, emotional, relational, sexual, and spiritual challenges that occur at the time of diagnosis and following surgery. We've shared our experiences, our struggles, the serious mistakes we've made, and the lessons we learned to equip you and guide you through this difficult and frightening journey.

We did not write this book to advocate, advance, or bash prostate surgery. The surgical option isn't the right choice for everyone. It is, however, the most heavily promoted and advertised treatment option.

All the advertising for robotic surgery is geared toward making you believe life will return to normal shortly after surgery. It is true that there are some fortunate men who experience an uneventful and rapid recovery from surgery. These men regain urinary control within days of their catheters being removed, and they regain their erectile function within days or weeks.

That's one possible outcome from surgery. It could be yours. We had a very different experience. We learned there are temporary and permanent life-altering consequences you and your partner will face after surgery. That's why we believe it is extremely important to visit a prostate cancer support group in person or to join an online support group.

This gives you the opportunity to meet with others who have dealt with the life-altering consequences of prostate surgery.

Since I (Rick) had a number of pre-existing urological issues prior to surgery, some of the difficulties we experienced were a result of my previous medical history rather than a direct result of surgery. For example, my urologist warned me it was possible I could be in the minority of men who would never regain urinary control. Within a week, I forgot about this warning. A few months after my surgery I was reminded of this conversation after I reread my notes from that appointment.

I think most men are shell-shocked when they receive the diagnosis of prostate cancer. It's common to forget very important information your doctors share with you. My advice is to make a list of questions prior to all your doctors' appointments. Have your spouse or a friend or family member accompany you. Take good notes or record the answers to your questions.

Prior to my surgery, I thought my prior professional training and experience as a medical social worker and Brenda's experience as a nurse would make this journey easier for us. I was wrong. I found coping with the aftermath of surgery extremely difficult. If you choose surgery as your treatment option, you'll find this book is filled with practical tips and information specific to surgery. If you choose another treatment option but want to know more about how the diagnosis of prostate cancer will impact your life and relationships, you will find many chapters very helpful.

At this point, you may feel all alone and isolated. According to the American Cancer Society, 241,740 men will receive a diagnosis of prostate cancer in 2012.[1] It's important early on to tap into the knowledge base of men who are further

---

1   http://www.cancer.org/Cancer/ProstateCancer/DetailedGuide/prostate-cancer-key-statistics

along in this journey. Reading this book is one way to gain some of that knowledge. Some men who are lost refuse to ask for directions, and I want to give them a special warning: the road you are traveling is treacherous. You will avoid many needless problems and suffering if you are wise enough to learn from those who've traveled farther along the road you are on. Would you prefer to drive a treacherous road blindfolded or with someone who is so familiar with the road he can warn you in advance when there are dangerous curves and potholes along your path?

If you choose surgery as your treatment option, there are many issues doctors gloss over or do not discuss at all. For example, even if surgery cures you of cancer, there is a high likelihood you will experience moderate to severe depression. It's doubtful you will be warned about or prepared for how to cope with post-surgical depression.

My wife and I faced many issues that affected us as individuals and as a couple. Recovering from the aftermath of surgery was difficult and highly stressful. It's not a journey couples should face by themselves.

Sadly, too often men shut down and keep their emotional struggles to themselves. To every man diagnosed with prostate cancer, believe me when I tell you support from your partner is vital. This book was written to help couples journey together. You'll find a number of questions at the end of most chapters. Choose the questions that are most important and relevant to you, and discuss them together. If you are members of a support group, bring the book with you and ask the group if they'd be willing to use the questions as topics to discuss together.

I wanted this book to speak to both men and women, so I asked my wife, Brenda, if she would write a few chapters to share her perspective on what it was like for her to go through this experience with me. She was willing to share her perspective, and her chapters can be found later in the book.

If you take away only one suggestion from this book, it should be this: *face this disease with a team rather than alone.* By making the commitment to read *I Left My Prostate in San Francisco—Where's Yours?,* you've added Brenda and me to your team. It's our prayer that our experiences, the questions we've provided for you to discuss, and the resources we share will make a difference in how you'll deal with your experiences with prostate cancer.

My wife and I believe it is privilege to take this journey with you. Therefore, we decided to share intimate details of our emotional struggles, our relational and sexual struggles, as well as our faith. We did this so you might feel more comfortable opening your life to your spouse and/or other members of your team.

Chapter 1

The Journey Begins

Each man has his own story how he received the diagnosis of prostate cancer. Usually it begins with a lump discovered on a digital exam or a sudden rise in our PSA. A PSA test measures the amount of a protein produced by the prostate. The PSA test has been widely used to screen men for prostate cancer. Starting at age forty, it is recommended that men have their PSA tested and a digital exam every year. I had both eight months prior to my office visit with my urologist on December 10, 2011. The sole purpose for this appointment was for me to obtain a prescription renewal. When I'm feeling healthy, going to the doctor and putting up with a long wait in the lobby seems like a colossal waste of time.

When my son Andy was eight years old, he had to wait a few hours to see an ear, nose, and throat doctor regarding a problem with his vocal cords. When the appointment was over, he said, "Dad, I came into this office as young boy, but we've been here so long I'm leaving as an old man." I never forgot Andy's perspective on waiting for doctors' appointments. When I entered the lobby, I was fifty-eight years old. It wouldn't take much waiting for me to leave as an old man.

As I looked at the many faces in the lobby, it was

obvious some of those people were suffering. I recalled how many times I'd been in that office suffering so badly that death would have been a welcome relief. Not this day—I was feeling great! I felt better than I had in years. I was both joyful and thankful to feel so healthy. I took some time to thank God for my current state of good health.

In the middle of those thoughts, I heard the nurse call my name. I was led to an office and told to wait for the doctor. My doctor came in, sat down, and said, "What brings you here today?"

I replied, "Doc, this is going to be the easiest appointment of your day. All you need to do is renew my prescription for Uroxatral and I'm outta here."

The doctor said, "I'm willing to do that, but since you're here, I'd like to check your prostate."

Alarm bells went off in my head. I wasn't due for another prostate exam for at least four months. Like most men, this is my least-favorite exam. I try to avoid it whenever possible. Today was no exception. So I said, "How about this? You give me the script today, and I'll schedule a prostate exam in four months."

I thought that was a reasonable request, and I expected the doctor to agree with my plan. I was unpleasantly surprised when he said he would not renew my prescription unless he checked my prostate. His response really ticked me off. I had come into the office specifically to get my prescription renewed. That's all I wanted.

I decided my doctor needed to learn I was a health-care consumer and he worked for me. There was no way I would be coaxed or threatened into a prostate exam. My plan was to storm out of the office, saying, "I'll see you in four months."

Before I could get up and put my plan into action, however, my wife chimed in with her opinion. Since my wife wasn't with me at the time, you may be curious as to how she managed to get her opinion heard.

Many years ago, I discovered I have two wives. My first wife is Brenda. We've been married for thirty-two years. She was at home at the time of the exam. However, my second wife, whose name happens to be Brenda, lives in my head. She can speak to me from anywhere. She bears a striking resemblance to the woman I married. In fact, they are one and the same person, except they reside in two different places. The Brenda in my head goes with me everywhere. There is no separating from her or going someplace she can't reach me. I wasn't surprised to hear the Brenda in my head offer her opinion on this matter.

Unfortunately for me, she had a different opinion about me receiving a prostate exam, and I knew why. Her eyes weren't about to bulge out of their sockets during the exam; mine were. Try as I might, I could not convince the Brenda in my head that walking out on this exam would be a good learning experience for my doctor. My wife happens to be an RN, which means the Brenda in my head is also an RN. If a doctor orders an exam, it's an RN's job to make sure the exam gets done. My doctor had just said I needed a prostate exam, so the Brenda in my head said, "Pull down your pants and assume the position."

The doctor must have thought I was crazy. There I was sitting in a chair, unable to respond to his request to get up and pull down my pants. I sat glued to the chair while I argued with the Brenda in my head. I was telling her there was no way I was going to have my prostate examined. I was quite certain the Brenda at home would be as ticked off as the Brenda in my head if I refused the exam. I asked myself if I really wanted to go home and explain to my wife that I was willing to suffer for four months without my prescription just to make a point. The Brenda in my head warned me not to come home without my prescription refilled. The warning was ominous, and I knew I'd just lost the argument. So I got up from the chair, pulled down my pants, leaned over the table, and gave the doctor the unspoken message: "Let the exam begin."

There was no way to predict or anticipate that the next five seconds would suddenly send a powerful tremor into my life. After the exam, my doctor explained he'd felt a suspicious lump. He went on to say I'd need an appointment for a biopsy. I couldn't believe what I had just heard. I had come into the office feeling great. All I wanted and expected was a prescription renewal.

Suddenly and unexpectedly I was facing the possibility I had prostate cancer. The fear I've felt when I've experienced a nightmare overwhelmed me. There was one difference: I knew this fear wouldn't fade away because this nightmare began while I was awake. Since part of me could not accept the possibility that I had prostate cancer, I developed a plan to avoid the biopsy. I asked the doctor if he'd order a PSA test. He agreed to do this. I went out to the reception area to schedule a biopsy. Scheduling the test did not mean I intended to have one; it meant I was going along to get along. Once I had my PSA score, I had every intention of canceling the biopsy. I was certain my PSA would show that the biopsy was totally unnecessary.

I was in a state of shock during the drive home from my exam. I couldn't escape a thought that kept playing in my mind like a broken record: "I might have prostate cancer." Each time that played in my head, I'd answer back, "That's impossible. I feel too healthy to have cancer."

On the way home, I wondered how to break this news to my wife. I knew there was no way she would hear the word *cancer,* and allow me to deny that possibility. The best I could hope for was a low PSA so I could talk Brenda into letting me postpone the biopsy for a year or two. After all, I had my prescription refill in my hand, and that was all I wanted when I'd scheduled my appointment.

I didn't want to go in for a biopsy. It would have been impossible to deny I had prostate cancer if a biopsy showed I did. As I thought about the possibility of receiving a diagnosis of cancer, two emotions became my constant companions: fear and anxiety.

Questions to Consider

1. What are your experiences with people who've been diagnosed with cancer?

2. What have those experiences led you to think and feel about cancer?

3. Has anyone in your family or circle of friends been diagnosed with prostate cancer?

4. What happened to him after he was diagnosed?

5. On a one-through-ten scale, with one being the lowest and ten being the highest level, rate:

   Your level of fear: _____.

   Your level of anxiety: _____.

6. What's your history with regard to how you have dealt with anxiety and fear in the past?

7. What's your history with your faith upholding you in times of crisis?

8. Who is available for support as you deal with the crisis?

9. What support do you need from your partner at this time?

Chapter 2

Losing My Judgment, Perhaps My Mind

Obtaining the results of my PSA test became vitally important. The right results would end the disturbingly recurrent thought, *I may have prostate cancer.* This sentence had been repeating in my mind every day, many times a day since the lump was discovered during my digital exam.

After four days, I called my urologist's office to obtain results of my PSA test. Here's a chronology of the events that almost landed me in jail, when all I wanted was my PSA score.

> Day 1: I called the urologist's office for my PSA results. They never called me back.

> Day 2: I asked the receptionist to leave the nurse a message to call me on my cell phone regarding my PSA score. I told her specifically that if I didn't pick up the phone to just give me my score. A few hours later, the nurse called me back. I was unable to pick up the phone. As soon as I had time, I called the message center. I expected to hear my PSA results. Instead I heard the nurse telling me to

call her back. I did so immediately, but she did not return my call, so day two passed without me receiving my PSA score.

Day 3: I called the office the moment it opened. Once again I asked the receptionist to tell the nurse to leave me my score on my cell phone whether I answer my phone or not. By mid-afternoon, I had not received a return phone call.

At that point, I got a flash of brilliance. I figured out a way to get my PSA score and get it immediately. I started thinking about buying a gun, going down to my doctor's office, pointing an unloaded gun at the receptionist, and asking, "Is this what it takes in order to get my PSA score?" As I thought this through, I imagined how it might end. In my mind's eye I saw my picture on the front page of the *Modesto Bee* (our local newspaper) of me being taken away in handcuffs, with the headline, "Man Driven to Desperation by Insensitive Medical Care." I *liked it!* No, I *loved it!* I thought it would make a great front-page story, and I'd be proud I was in it.

At that point I decided to discuss this idea with the Brenda in my head before I discussed it with the Brenda I live with. The Brenda in my head was wonderfully supportive. She was also wise. She suggested I buy a toy gun. She pointed out how much money I would save by purchasing a toy gun. In addition, she said, I'd probably face reduced charges and less jail time if I used a toy gun.

I was startled to discover how much smarter the Brenda in my head was compared to me. With her advice, I was certain the Brenda I lived with would support my plan. I was unpleasantly surprised when the Brenda I married didn't react the same way as the Brenda in my head. The Brenda I married was horrified that I liked the idea of buying a toy gun, making front-page news, and going to jail just to get the results from my PSA test, without any further delays. That's how desperate I felt. In fact, I thought I'd be a media hero because I was exposing the damaging effects of insensitive and unresponsive medical practitioners.

I seriously hate it when I think I have a truly great idea but then my wife comes along to tell me my idea stinks. As if that's not bad enough, it turned out she was right. Anyone who's been married more than a day can identify with this gripe. At that point, I was still insisting my plan was brilliant. The Brenda I live with asked me to think of a better idea. Like there was one!

That's the teacher in Brenda. She didn't want to give me a better idea; she wanted me to come up with one myself. I couldn't. I was certain my idea was the best idea possible. Fortunately for me, the office called me a short time later and gave me the results of my PSA test. Looking back, it's frightening to realize how desperate I was and what I considered doing to get my results. My PSA was 5.8. This was almost double my previous PSA level of eight months earlier. A disturbing mathematical formula came to my mind. It went like this:

A palpable lump + a doubling of PSA in eight months = prostate cancer

All my attempts at denial were shattered when I received the results of my PSA test. I went from denial to 100 percent certainty I had prostate cancer. I was convinced the biopsy was simply a formality and would only confirm what I already knew. The idea was terrifying, but I still managed to find a way to deny this frightening reality. I began to hope the biopsy would show a benign growth. I tried to convince myself the sudden rise in my PSA was a result of my digital exam performed before my PSA test. This wasn't based on wishful thinking; PSA scores often rise as a result of a digital exam. There was some factual basis I could use to support my denial, but the mathematical formula kept relentlessly repeating in my mind. I began to seesaw back and forth. One moment I was convinced I had cancer, and in the next, I attributed the jump in PSA to a benign growth combined with a digital exam. I became as desperate to have the biopsy results as I had been to obtain my PSA. My urologist's office was so backed up that my biopsy was scheduled thirty days out. Then the only appointment they had to discuss the results of my biopsy was two weeks after the test.

It was clear to me the urology office I'd been with for almost thirty years had a long history of moving slowly. It had taken three days with multiple phone calls to get my PSA results. Now they wanted me to wait thirty days for a biopsy and then two weeks more for the results. This was unacceptable. I was dealing with the terrifying possibility that I had prostate cancer. The fact that I was dealing with a practice that to me seemed cold, impersonal, and slow added to my suffering. There was no way I could have coped with waiting six weeks to find out if I had cancer.

Brenda and I decided it was time to put together a new medical team— a team that would schedule tests and get the results back to me on a timely basis. Brenda and I took this issue to God in prayer.

A few days later, a urologist who had treated me for a urinary disease seven years earlier came to mind. I called his office and discovered he would be willing to take me on as a patient. They were able to get me in two weeks earlier than I was scheduled for my biopsy at the other practice. I wanted my first exam to be my biopsy. This was an unusual request. At first it was refused. This urologist wanted to use the first appointment to perform a digital exam and then decide for himself whether I needed a biopsy. After discussing this with my wife, we realized this could add an additional few weeks to wait for a biopsy.

I called the office back. I explained that I was certain I had prostate cancer and it was important to me to have my biopsy as quickly as possible. I told them I'd get a copy of my last exam and that I already had the antibiotics at home, as well as the enema kit, both of which I needed to use before the biopsy. I asked if they could schedule the digital exam and my biopsy on the same day. The doctor was kind enough to agree to this plan. This was all the evidence I needed that it was time to switch to a team that would meet my needs as a prostate cancer patient.

I called my original urologist's office, canceled my biopsy, and made arrangements for my medical records to be transferred to the new urologist's office. I'm a person who likes to save time and do things efficiently. It was inconvenient to drive seventy miles round trip for my urological care, but there was an important lesson I needed to learn quickly. When it comes to obtaining lifesaving treatment, if you are wise, you *must* give up the idea of comfort, familiarity, and convenience. Switching to a different medical team was the first step toward entering a new world that involved going places I didn't want to go to get tests and treatments I'd rather not have experienced in order to fight and treat a disease I didn't want to have.

By making these new arrangements, I was able to move my biopsy up by two weeks and the time I'd have to spend waiting for the results by a little more than a week.

Questions to Consider

1. What was it that led your doctor to order a biopsy for you?

2. How did this news affect you?

3. What do you want to know about biopsies before you have one?

4. Would you allow your fear about this procedure stop you from obtaining it?

5. If so, what can be done to help you conquer your fears?

Chapter 3

Preparing for Your Biopsy

Some men are so afraid of this procedure that they will delay or refuse to get a biopsy. The more I read about the procedure, the more I understood why. The idea of a needle puncturing my rectum multiple times brought a significant sense of dread into my life. There are a few different ways this procedure is performed, but the preparation is similar.

Your urologist will need to know what medications you are taking that increase the risk of bleeding. This will include prescriptions and all over-the-counter supplements. You will be asked to stop taking these for a few days before your biopsy. On the day of your appointment, you will give yourself an enema at home, and you will also take an antibiotic at a specified time before your biopsy.

I am not a fan of pain. Additionally, it's been my experience that when a physician tells me, "This will feel like a little poke," I prepare myself to feel the pain of being stabbed with a six-inch blade that will be twisted and turned before it's pulled out. Since my biggest concern was how much pain I'd experience, I decided to find out from men who've had a biopsy just how painful the procedure was. I wanted the real scoop on the level of pain I'd experience for this procedure.

I went on-line to ask men whether their biopsy was a painful experience. A few men found the procedure extremely painful. The larger majority found their biopsy mildly to moderately uncomfortable. I read one blog that compared a prostate biopsy to getting sodomized by a knitting needle. After reading those words, my fear about the procedure escalated from mild anxiety to full-blown terror. Sometimes what you read on the Internet makes things worse than they really are. Something constructive came about through my research. I resolved I would not be in the group of men who received nothing for pain control. Whatever was available, I wanted it. There was no doubt that if I had my choice at that point I would have preferred to be unconscious.

On biopsy day, I learned I was having a transrectal biopsy. Many urologists give an injection of Lidocaine to dull pain, but others do not. I wanted the injection, and it was offered to me. The good news was that the Lidocaine injections effectively dull the pain of the biopsy. The bad news was that I found the injections to reduce the pain to be painful. I suppose that's why some urologists skip the Lidocaine.

My memories about this procedure are clear, vivid, and accurate. My urologist showed me a spring-loaded device with a two-foot needle that would penetrate my rectum and tear away tissue from the prostate. My wife claims the needle was only a few inches long. You can choose who you are going to believe—the guy who felt a two-foot needle penetrating his rectum, or my wife, who happens to be an RN. I felt brief stabs of pain that quickly went away.

The exam takes approximately fifteen minutes. The biopsy is only the beginning of being poked, prodded, and stabbed on the journey to a prostatectomy. If I had to go through a biopsy again, I would ask to be sedated. With conscious sedation, you will be able to speak, respond to commands, and communicate your level of comfort or pain. This level of sedation would totally eliminate the pain associated with this procedure. On a one-to-ten scale, with ten being the most pain, I'd rate the procedure a four or five.

If your fear about this procedure is sky high, insist on sedation. There are some urologists who will refuse this request because they believe it is inappropriate or unnecessary. Pain is always less painful when someone else is feeling the pain. Not everyone needs sedation, but if you want it, find an urologist who will respect your need for this level of pain control.

After your biopsy, there will be some expected side effects, and there is one specific side effect you may experience but not be warned about. Here are two you will be warned about:

1. Blood in your urine or rectal bleeding that could occur for a few days.

2. Blood in the semen for a few weeks and for some a few months.

Seeing blood-red semen was somewhat of a shock to my wife and me. Truthfully, I was grossed out, and so was my wife. There is also one side effect that's considered so rare it may not be mentioned in the biopsy consent form you signed. Naturally, it happened to me. I became temporarily impotent. Rather than calling my urologist, I went online and typed in "impotence after a prostate biopsy." I found a number of articles and studies that confirmed this as a possible side effect.

I personally believe temporary impotence is not as rare as doctors think. I can't help but wonder how many men like me experience this but don't report it to anyone. Once I learned that impotence is a temporary side effect that lasts two weeks, I waited, and my sexual function returned. If it happens to you, don't worry. However, if your sexual function does not return within two weeks, you should call your urologist. After an adverse reaction to the injection prior to my bone scan and my experience with impotence after the biopsy, whenever a doctor said to me, "This rarely happens," I became convinced it was going to happen to me. More often than not, it did.

There are issues you can discuss with your urologist before you have your biopsy:

- ❒ The type of biopsy that will be performed.
- ❒ The type of pain control your doctor typically offers. If you want to be sedated, make sure your urologist knows this in advance and agrees to it.
- ❒ The odds your biopsy will not detect cancer present in your prostate.
- ❒ How and where you will receive the results from your biopsy.

Some urologists tell their patients there is no need for pain management to perform a biopsy. Having experienced a biopsy, I disagree. It's my advice you meet with your urologist to find a mutually agreeable plan for pain control.

It will take a few days for your urologist to get the results back from your biopsy. I did not want to be called in to the office for the results. I wanted to get them in the privacy of my home. My urologist agreed to call me at home with the results within four days after my biopsy.

Questions to Consider

1. How do you want to receive the results of your biopsy, by phone or with an office visit?

2. Who will provide you with emotional support as you wait for the results?

3. Discuss how you will think, feel, and what you'll fear if you receive the news you have prostate cancer?

Chapter 4

I Have Prostate Cancer

On Sunday, January 16, in the early morning hours, my phone rang. It was my urologist. As soon as I heard the tone of his voice, I had a sense the news I was about to hear would not be good. I asked him to wait a moment before giving me the results. I wanted to receive the news with my wife. She was sleeping at the time. I ran up the stairs, put my cell phone on speaker, and woke my wife. My biopsy results confirmed my greatest fear. I had prostate cancer.

Even though I had anticipated this news, it was no less devastating to receive it. Once I heard the word *cancer*, I stopped hearing the additional information my urologist was sharing. I had to ask him to wait until I got a pen and paper so I could write down the information. I knew if I didn't do that, I would not remember a thing.

Depending on your style of coping, you may have read extensively about prostate cancer prior to receiving the results. From the other direction, it's possible you decided not to read anything until it became necessary. There's no right way to cope. Once you receive your biopsy results, it's important for you to understand your Gleason scores. In 1966 Dr. Gleason discovered a way to classify cancer cells in order to determine the aggressiveness of prostate cancer.

It is important for you to ask the doctor who provides you with your Gleason scores to take the time to explain what your scores mean in terms of the aggressiveness of the cancer cells in your prostate. Your biopsy results are your initial scores taken from a small sample of your prostate. If you choose surgery, you will receive a second pathology report. It's possible your Gleason scores will be the same, more serious, or less serious than the Gleason scores you received from your biopsy. After my biopsy, cancer was found in four cores. My Gleason scores were 3+4 in three cores and 3+3 in the other. My urologist said 3+4 was moderately aggressive.

When the word *aggressive* is attached to the word *cancer*, the words *mild* or *moderate* become meaningless. As a person with cancer, all you hear and all that matters is that you have an aggressive cancer. From an emotional and intellectual level, it's the words *aggressive cancer* you will react to. My world was rocked with an earthquake that registered ten on the Richter scale. Remember, the person receiving the diagnosis is not the only one experiencing this quake. Your spouse, your children, and those who love you will have their worlds rocked in this quake as well.

Here's a partial list of things that are shaken in the quake:

◆ Your sense of good health
◆ Your sense of safety
◆ Your long-term plans for your future
◆ Your financial well being
◆ Your predictability of life
◆ Your identity
◆ Your faith
◆ Your friendships
◆ Your priorities
◆ Your values

♦ Your use of time

♦ The importance of your work

Take time to talk to your partner so each of you can share your reactions to receiving this awful news. I want to offer you some reassurance. If you've been diligent with yearly PSA testing and digital exams, there is an excellent chance your prostate cancer was found early. Prostate cancer is a very treatable form of cancer, especially when it's found in the early stages.

You have much to do and learn so you can decide the most effective way to treat your cancer.

Questions to Consider

1. How will you learn about the various ways to treat prostate cancer?

2. Are there doctors from different specialties, radiologists, surgeons, etc, you need to consult with?

3. Can you be treated locally or would you prefer to travel to a specialized prostate cancer treatment center?

4. Are there further tests needed such as a bone scan or ultrasound?

Chapter 5

Bones Scanned

There are differing opinions in the medical field about whether every man with prostate cancer needs a bone scan prior to surgery. I'd been experiencing bone pain for months before I received a diagnosis of prostate cancer. I'm certain my complaint of pain in my bones was the primary reason my urologist ordered a bone scan.

Unlike the biopsy, I had no sense of physical dread about taking this test. I knew it would be painless. The only serious dread I had was about the results. I was afraid my bone pain was a symptom of bone cancer, which is a common occurrence with advanced prostate cancer. I expected this procedure to be incident free. It didn't turn out that way. Before a bone scan, a small amount of a radioactive dye is injected into your vein. After the injection, you will be told to come back for the scan in a few hours. After my injection, I was told to go home and given a specific time to return for the scan. I left the hospital, got in my car, and started to drive home.

Within a minute or two, I felt the most intense need to urinate I'd ever experienced. I turned my car around and sped right back to the hospital. Once I was in the parking lot, I had to run into the lobby to immediately reach the bathroom. I was glad I made it before I had an embarrassing accident. After that experience, I was afraid to get back into my car to drive home, so I sat in the lobby for a few minutes waiting to see if a sudden urge would overtake me again. It didn't, so I decided to strategically plan my five-mile drive home.

I wanted to be certain I'd have the ability to stop at gas stations along the way in case I needed to make an emergency bathroom stop. I had intended to go back to work, but there was no way that was going to be possible. I needed to stay home and have immediate access to my bathroom. This was an example of something I experienced many times throughout my journey with prostate cancer, and it was frustrating. Why didn't someone say to me, *"There is a possibility you'll experience an intense need to urinate after the injection. It would be a good idea to stay in the lobby for fifteen minutes so you can use the bathroom a few times if necessary before taking the drive home"?*

I don't understand why, as prostate cancer patients, we receive very little preparation for the things we are going to experience along the way. Unfortunately, this was the first of many times in this journey where I would not receive an appropriate warning or information. Adequate preparation increases the likelihood of success for any journey. As I share my journey with you, it's my goal to prepare you for the many issues that will arise so you will be well prepared for the road ahead. The drive back from the scan was incident free because my bladder was empty.

The bone scan itself was easy. I got to see myself as a skeleton. I had two powerful impressions. First, I noticed my love handles didn't show, so I looked much skinnier and more handsome as a skeleton. From my perspective, I hadn't looked that good in decades. My second thought was I wanted a copy of the picture of myself so I could show off. I was so pleased with how good I looked that I wanted to get a poster-size picture so I could use myself as a Halloween decoration. I thought it would be so cool to display a skeleton at Halloween and say to everyone who saw it, "That's not any old skeleton; that's me!" I was serious when I asked the tech if there was a way I could buy a blown-up image of myself as a skeleton. When he said no, I was disappointed.

It took a while for my bladder to settle down after the test, which was why I could not return to work for the rest of the day. I intended to enjoy the next two days I had to wait before I'd receive the news of whether the prostate cancer (PC) had spread into my bones. There were some moments of fear as well. It was a great relief when the results of my bone scan came back clear. I didn't have cancer in my bones. Some men will not be as fortunate. They will receive the terrible news that PC has spread to their bones. This news is not a death sentence. There is an amazing amount of research and treatments available to fight cancer in the bone.

To every man who receives this awful news, it's my suggestion that you consult with a specialist at a research facility or hospital that specializes in the treatment of advanced prostate cancer. If it means driving a few hundred miles, I think it would be worth your time and effort to do this. If I had received the news that cancer had spread to my bones, I would have contacted a major treatment center to determine whether I could participate in a clinical trial using experimental drugs.

Questions to Consider if You Have Metastasis to Your Bones

1. What are your greatest fears about this diagnosis? Discuss this with your partner, and family.

2. Have you shared some of these concerns with the physician in charge of your treatment? If not, why not?

3. Have you thought about a consult with a specialist? If so, do you need a referral?

4. What information do you need to help you treat/ fight advanced prostate cancer?

Questions to Consider if You Don't Have Metastasis to Your Bones

1. Once you've received the results of your biopsy and the bone scan, It is up to you to decide how to treat your cancer. How will you make that decision?

2. Make a list of pros and cons for choosing the surgical option.

3. Do you want to speak to other men who've gone through surgery? If so, do you want to do that face to face, or online? Take the steps you need to take in order to meet with men who've had surgery.

If you choose surgery, read every chapter. If you've ruled out surgery, some of this book will no longer be relevant to your experiences. However, there are many chapters that can help you along the way, such as Sharing the News, Celebrate, Good Comfort, Miserable Comfort, and others which apply to every man who is diagnosed with prostate cancer.

No matter which form of treatment you choose, do not skip Chapter 15 regarding in-network or out–of-network insurance policies—reading that chapter could save you thousands of dollars.

Chapter 6

Sharing the News

Deciding how, when, where, and with whom to share the news of my prostate cancer was not an easy task. There are no guidelines or protocol for doing this. When I first shared the news with other people, I had no idea what to expect. Obviously, most people were as shocked as I was. What images come to your mind when you think of someone with cancer? Maybe you think of someone who lost all of his or her hair. I've been bald for twenty years now. Maybe you think of someone who is severely underweight. I'm carrying at least twenty pounds more than I should be, mostly around the middle. Maybe you think of someone with cancer as someone who moves slowly, with an obvious lack of energy. I'm from New York. I do everything quickly. If I had to drive to my own execution, I'd be in the left lane, passing everyone in order to get there as soon as possible. I was still capable of living at that speed. The fact is, I didn't look or feel like someone who had cancer. That's what made the news so unbelievable to me and often to those I told.

The people who had the most intense reactions were, as a general rule, those who had a friend or family member who had been diagnosed with cancer. For example, after I told someone I had prostate cancer, the first words back to me were, "I'm so sorry; my father died of prostate cancer."

I expected to share the news and immediately receive comforting words back. Instead I felt more anxious and afraid. After a number of these experiences, I had to take a break from telling people the news face to face.

I told my pastor early on about my cancer, but I asked him not to announce the news to the congregation. He was both wise and kind enough to know we needed prayer, so he found a way to honor my request and still have our church family praying for us. Each week he'd ask the congregation to keep a friend of his (me) who had been diagnosed with cancer in their prayers.

Some people prefer to use a blog or social media to share information with their friends or family. That saves you from repeating the same information over and over again. I found e-mail to be a safe way to share the news. I own two sandwich shops. I told each of my managers the news face to face. I posted a letter at both my locations to inform the staff. I invited all my employees to speak with me about it if they so desired.

There were a few life lessons necessary to learn before I was going to resume personally sharing the news. First, it was important to take into account how the news would impact the person I was telling. Receiving the news that a friend or family member was diagnosed with cancer is traumatic to the person receiving it. I was so preoccupied with my fears that I didn't consider what it would be like for the person receiving the news from me.

Second, almost every person I told about my prostate cancer wanted to share an experience they had with cancer. Most of those stories had a similar ending—someone they knew or loved died from cancer. Hearing these stories increased my levels of fear and anxiety, which was the opposite result of what I hoped to receive. I wanted to feel comfort or feel better as a result of sharing the news. Instead, I got ticked off that I had to listen to a story about someone else who had cancer, especially when the end of the story involved that person dying.

At some point, I gained a valuable understanding about the stories people were sharing. I had assumed they were ignoring my plight and changing the subject by talking about their own experiences. I couldn't have been more wrong. I learned it was important to pay close attention to the story someone was sharing. This wasn't a case of someone changing the subject or ignoring my story; it was all about my news triggering the memory of a relevant experience. The story they shared provided me with an understanding of how they were feeling about the news they had just received. Since most of the stories were about people who had died, I realized the people I shared the news with had the same association I had when I first heard the word cancer, and that was death.

The people who told me those stories were afraid I was going to die from prostate cancer. Hearing the news that someone close to you was diagnosed with cancer brings up what I'll call an existential fear. I know all about this fear. So does every man diagnosed with prostate cancer. It is frightening to come to grips with how fragile our good health is. We don't like to think that one minute we can be healthy and the next minute discover we weren't healthy at all but in fact have a potentially life-threatening disease.

When you hear the news that someone you know and love had been unexpectedly diagnosed with cancer, your own sense of safety or good health is threatened as well. You think, *If that could happen to him, then something like that could happen to me.* Once I understood how traumatic it was for my friends and family to hear I had prostate cancer, I realized it was unrealistic to expect them to provide any comfort when I shared the news. Comfort would come later. Additionally, I stopped feeling angry, hurt, neglected, or frustrated as people shared their personal experiences with cancer with me. In fact, I paid close attention because I understood the stories they shared were the filter they were using to process and understand the news of my cancer. Remember this: if you find yourself disappointed, neglected, hurt, or angry when you share the news, try to remember how traumatic it was for the person receiving it. He or she may need your comfort!

My first opportunity to apply what I learned came when one of my staff members asked me how I was feeling. She was particularly worried about the amount of pain I was experiencing. I thought that was an odd query because I had never experienced any pain. So rather than answering her question, I asked about her experience with cancer. She told me all about her mom, who died a slow and painful death as a result of bone cancer. Since that was her experience, she was expecting me to be in the same pain as her mother. Additionally, she was expecting me to die in the near future. Once I understood her experiences, we discussed the differences between my cancer and her mother's. This conversation went well for both of us.

It took me almost two months after receiving my biopsy results to gain the insights and skills I needed to be ready to share my diagnosis with my church family. With those insights and understanding in place, I called my pastor. At the next worship service, he announced the news. I was ready to hear reactions from other people. Once this news was shared, we began to receive cards, phone calls, prayer, and other support. It is truly a blessing to be part of a church family when you are facing a traumatic event like cancer.

As I shared the news, I found myself educating men about prostate cancer. I'd ask men when they'd had their last PSA or digital exam. A few men made appointments with their doctors after I shared my story.

Sharing the news with your children is different than sharing the news with other people. How you share depends upon the ages of your children. Since prostate cancer usually hits men in their fifties and older, most of the time children have reached at least their teens when you receive your diagnosis. There may be grandchildren you'd want to tell as well. If there are young children or grandchildren involved, my suggestion is to keep your explanations simple. Say, "Grandpa is sick and will need to go to the hospital to get better." That's as detailed as you need to get.

I have three sons in their twenties and a teenage daughter. I believe it's a good idea to keep your children informed during each phase you go through. My first discussion involved telling my children that a doctor had felt a lump in my prostate, and I was referred for a biopsy to determine whether I had cancer. Once I received my biopsy results, I told my children I had cancer and it was mildly aggressive. I explained that I chose surgery as the way to treat my cancer. I felt it was important to speak with each child individually. I wanted to provide each of our children the opportunity to ask questions and express their concerns, thoughts, or feelings without their other siblings present. If my children were frightened in any way, they chose to keep their fears to themselves.

There's something else I highly recommend you share with your children in addition to the news you were diagnosed with cancer. Share your love for each of your children and grandchildren. Let them all know how much they mean to you. Don't forget to tell your partner this as well. If there is a history of anger, bitterness, or unforgiveness, become a peacemaker wherever possible. Be the first to offer forgiveness. You have at least six weeks before your surgery to express your love and bring healing to estranged relationships wherever that's possible. Use that time in the service of love.

There is another important issue involving prostate cancer that every man should discuss with his biological sons. I chose to wait until I recovered from surgery and regained urinary control before bringing this issue up. There is a hereditary component to developing prostate cancer. Once you've been diagnosed, there is a higher probability your sons may develop prostate cancer as well. After age forty, it's important for them to be vigilant about yearly digital exams and PSA testing. It's not only important to share this with your sons; their doctors should be made aware of this medical history as well.

Here's a list of issues I believe are important to address before you have surgery. These tasks may frighten you, but they are important and should be taken care of.

- Do you have a will? If not, see an attorney and make one.

- Do you have life insurance? If so, make sure your wife/children know the location of your policy.

- If you knew you wouldn't see your family ever again, what would you tell them?

- Make sure your wife, partner, or a family member has medical power of attorney.

- Prepare an advance directive, which makes your wishes known should you become incapacitated. Make sure a copy of this directive is in your medical files prior to surgery.

Questions to Consider

1. How will you break the news you have prostate cancer to

   A. Your children?

   B. Your grandchildren?

   C. Your extended family?

   D. Your friends?

   E. Your religious community?

   F. Your co-workers?

   G. Your boss?

2. Are there people you'd prefer to break this news to in writing?

3. Are there people you don't want to know about your diagnosis at this point in time?

4. How will you keep those who you want to share the news with informed?

5. Are there any other things you need to say or do prior to your surgery?

6. Is there anyone you'd like to appoint to share the news and updates of your condition?

Chapter 7

Laughing Is Good for the Soul

A merry heart makes a cheerful
countenance.—Proverbs 15:13

The concepts I'm about to share are things I wish I'd understood earlier in my journey. Depending on your current level of anxiety or fear, the next few chapters may appear out of place in a book about prostate cancer. There are many things along this journey that you could find humorous. In addition, there are ways to bring humor into your circumstances. I was surprised I could find so many things worth celebrating. If you are able to follow the suggestions in next few chapters about laughter and celebration, I believe you can reduce the severity and duration of post-surgical depression. You'll also have the ability to deal with relationship issues more effectively.

Finding positive ways to use humor will make a huge difference in how you cope with prostate cancer. One of the first things I did following my diagnosis was to go online and look for jokes about prostate cancer. Here's one I found extremely funny: A man goes in for a prostate exam. His urologist performs a digital exam. He finds a suspicious lump and tells the man he could have prostate cancer. The man asks his urologist if he will repeat the exam using another finger. The urologist replies, "Why should I do that?" The man says, "Because I'd like a second opinion."

I can't describe how healthy and beneficial it was when I was able to laugh about prostate cancer. At many points in the journey I focused my attention on things that would make me laugh. Here are a few of those humorous events. Some of these events occurred after my surgery.

The first time I purchased a case of diapers at Costco was traumatic. I didn't want the cashier to think the diapers were for me. I developed a plan while I was waiting in line. As the cashier began to ring up the diapers, I planned to ask my wife, "Honey, do you think those diapers will fit my dad?" There were two problems with my plan. First, my father died more than twenty years ago. Second, I thought of the plan while I was in front of the cashier. Therefore, I wasn't able to ask my wife to go along with my idea. I was terrified if I asked my wife that question, she'd say, "Honey, those aren't for your dad; he died long ago. Those diapers are for you."

Since that outcome would have been more humiliating than buying the diapers, I gave up on that plan. Sometimes we can come up with amazing ways to lie to ourselves to protect ourselves from humiliation. Since my first plan could have backfired, I lied to myself. I decided there was no way the cashier would ever think the diapers were for me because I looked much too young to need them. Sadly, when I got home and looked at myself in the mirror, staring back at me I saw a bald man with gray sideburns who certainly looked old enough to wear diapers. I realized the cashier would have had every reason to assume those diapers were mine.

Eventually my sanity returned, and I realized the cashier was so busy that the reality was she never even gave a thought as to who would be wearing those adult diapers. Looking back at the whole incident brought me peals of laughter. After my embarrassment at Costco, I decided to order additional diapers and pads online.

I don't know how I ordered so many pads, but when the first shipment arrived, I had ordered a ridiculous number of cases of pads. I probably could have supplied every woman in Modesto with pads for a month. I needed to find a way to share my pads, so I brought my teenage daughter into the room where I stored my cache. I prepared myself to experience a father-daughter moment. I said to her, "Kate, my pads are your pads; use them any time you'd like." The last thing I expected to see was my daughter rolling her eyes at me. To top it off, she said, "Daddy, you are so gross!" She quickly left the room. I learned the hard way that sharing pads isn't a father-daughter thing. There was such a gap between what I hoped would happen and what actually happened. I thought my error in judgment was hilarious.

One day I could not find my electric razor. I was certain I'd accidentally thrown it into the outside garbage pail. At the time I was unshaven, wearing my pajamas, and in a diaper which reeked from urine. Desperate to find my razor, I stuck my head deep into our garbage pail. Suddenly, I became fearful that a police officer driving by might see me rummaging through the garbage. I realized there was no way I could convince an officer I was conducting a search in my own driveway. I became so afraid of this possibility, I ran back to the house to clean up in order to safely resume the search for my razor. When I made it upstairs, I asked my wife what she would have told a police officer who knocked at our door to ask her if I lived there. My wife quickly replied, "I'd tell him I never saw you before in my life." Unshaven, in a diaper smelling of urine, it was a gift to laugh together at the absurdity of that imaginary scenario and my current state of dishevelment.

When I was at UCSF for the first consult to learn about penile injections, I wanted music to help me pass the time as I compressed the injection site. My nurse practitioner asked me what music I wanted. A song title immediately came to mind. It was "You Raise Me Up." So there I was sitting on the table with my pants hanging off my ankles. I had suffered the trauma of injecting a needle into my penis. My fear and embarrassment were sky high, yet all of us were cracking up. Laughter filled the room. We talked about piping that song through all the rooms used for penile injections, as well as in the surgery suite when the surgeons were working with the nerve bundles. Our laughter brought my fear and anxiety about my sticking needles into my penis to manageable levels. I was delighted to know I could share a laugh seconds after I'd had a needle stuck into my penis.

Pets can play a key role on the road to recovery. My dog, Teddy, was a wonderful source of comfort and laughter. During one of my walks with Teddy, I became obsessed with the question of how he would react if I opened up my catheter bag and put some of my urine over a spot where he'd just peed. I thought it could be a bonding experience. It would be the first (and last time) my dog and I would pee outside together. On one particular walk, I couldn't control this urge any longer. I reached for my catheter drain and planned to carry out the deed. My wife, who accompanied us on the walk, saw what I was about to do and said, "Don't you dare!" I suppose that was a good thing. If any of my neighbors saw me do this, how could I explain myself? What if they reported me to the police? Under those circumstances, I'm certain my wife would be in agreement with the decision to have me hauled off to the county mental health hospital for a psychiatric evaluation. I'm glad I heeded my wife's warning and skipped the bonding with Teddy.

A few weeks later, Teddy found a way to do something similar to me. After my catheter was pulled, I was using the bathroom every hour. For some odd reason, Teddy began following me into the bathroom. If I tried to close the door to keep him out, he'd scratch on the door and howl as if I were killing him. Eventually, I gave in to his distress and kept the door open so he could join me anytime he wanted. No matter what he was doing, if I went into the bathroom, Teddy was there in an instant. As I attempted to start a flow, Teddy would just sit there and watch. At first I thought this was very weird. Soon I considered him a cheerleader. I enjoyed his presence and thought of him as a great source of support.

After the first few weeks of following me into the bathroom, Teddy began visiting the bathroom on his own in order to pee by the toilet. It was as if he were saying to me, "I've seen you do this so many times now I'm going to do this too." The fact that Teddy and I were both using the bathroom to pee was funny. It wasn't funny having to clean and deodorize the bathroom floor, though. It became necessary to limit Teddy's access to the bathroom to the times I'd be in there. I also stopped him from smelling the toilet after I urinated. Within a few days, he stopped peeing in the bathroom. A year after surgery, Teddy still follows me into the bathroom every time I go, and I'm glad for his company. Thankfully, he stopped using the bathroom to pee.

There were many other wonderful times of laughter. I suggest you not only find places to laugh, I think it's a great idea to rent comedies. Spend as much time as you can laughing. If you have friends who make you laugh, make sure they are frequent guests in your home before and after surgery. Don't miss a single opportunity to laugh.

Questions to Consider

1. What activities do you do together as a couple that you both enjoy? Plan to do these things before and after surgery.

2. What things bring you laughter? Make a list, and plan to do things that make you laugh.

3. What things bring you comfort? Plan to do some of these things.

4. What friends and family do you have whose company you enjoy? Plan to have them visit you during your recovery.

5. What activities feed your soul? Make sure you make time to do these activities.

Chapter 8

Celebrate!

We associate celebrations with joyful occasions, such as birthdays, anniversaries, or weddings and special achievements like graduation. That's why the notion of celebrating anything associated with prostate cancer may sound ridiculous. Did I really want to celebrate that I learned to live without leaks by changing my diaper fifteen times a day? Yes! Celebrating every success was important. It was also funny. Never in my life did I expect to celebrate anything related to living in diapers. But I did.

There are milestones related to the diagnosis and treatment of prostate cancer that are worth celebrating. To celebrate means you will take time from your day to give thanks and/or take some time to do something special, fun, or entertaining because you crossed a milestone.

How you choose to celebrate is up to you. The phase you are in may limit the ways in which you can or want to celebrate. You will have more freedom to celebrate pre-surgery than you will immediately following surgery. I made myself a list of twenty-five things to celebrate. I hope you will use my list and add to it as you focus your attention on some of the good things that will happen to you on the path of your recovery.

Here are some things you can celebrate:

♦ We live in an age where the doctors are able to recommend that you have a biopsy. Years ago only men with advanced or terminal prostate cancer received treatment.

♦ You made it through your biopsy. (Not everyone can say he survived after his rectum was poked with a two-foot needle!)

♦ The fact that you have many different options to treat your prostate cancer. (Once you've received the diagnosis, this one might be difficult.)

♦ When you decide on a treatment option.

♦ When you've found the right surgeon to treat you.

♦ Your homecoming. You made it through surgery, and now you are back home.

♦ Having your catheter removed. Even though this event can bring on many difficult months of urinary incontinence, this is an important step toward healing.

♦ When you've learned how to manage pads.

♦ When a prayer is answered.

♦ When a friend or an acquaintance reaches out to you.

♦ If you received good news from the pathology report.

♦ You can have radiation or chemotherapy if your pathology report shows you need additional treatment.

♦ Any movement of God you see in your circumstances.

♦ When your experiences can be used to help others.

♦ Your first date after surgery.

♦ Your first orgasm. (This can happen without an erection.)

♦ Your mate's first orgasm post-surgery.

♦ Staying dry at night.

♦ Any reduction in the number of pads you use daily.

♦ When your leaking is limited to stress incontinence.

♦ Your first erection, whether it's with a pump, ED medication, a suppository, or by injection.

♦ Your first erection without artificial means. (This could take eighteen to twenty-four months.)

♦ When your fear of dying from prostate cancer lessens or vanishes.

♦ The results of your first post-surgery PSA test.

Chapter 9

Thirteen Ways to Celebrate

Here are some suggestions for celebrating; some are geared to post-surgery.

- ➢ Plan a romantic weekend getaway. Do this one prior to surgery and again a second time post-surgery, when you feel ready to enjoy traveling and getting away.
- ➢ Go out for your favorite meal.
- ➢ Order your favorite takeout and eat it at home.
- ➢ Rent a movie.
- ➢ Take your dog for a walk. Invite your partner too!
- ➢ Plan a romantic evening at home.
- ➢ Make time to enjoy a favorite activity—going to a concert, play, or movie.
- ➢ Make time to enjoy a hobby—camping, fishing, sports, etc.
- ➢ Take time to pray and find something you can express gratitude toward a blessing God has given to you.
- ➢ Throw a "grateful to be alive party."- Invite friends and/or family over for an evening of fun.

➢ Express an attitude of gratitude toward your partner for all the help and support you receive.

➢ Do something special with your children or grandchildren.

➢ Take a stroll down memory lane.-Get out old pictures. Recall the meaningful, memorable, highlights of your life. Enjoy these memories.

Add your ideas to this list.

Use the space below to write some of your own ways to celebrate your milestones.

Celebrating in general maintains the attitude of gratitude. If you are able to maintain your sense of gratitude, it will serve as an antidote to depression. Celebrating milestones is a reminder to remain thankful for the incremental progress you make as you recover from surgery. Celebrating acts of kindness doesn't take much effort. Coping with people who disappoint you isn't as easy.

Chapter 10

Be Careful with Great Expectations

At a time when I was feeling extremely vulnerable and frightened, I was pleasantly and unpleasantly surprised by the reactions of the people I knew. There will be some people who will surprise you with words or acts of kindness and comfort. Others will either hurt or disappoint you. Your relationships may change on the basis of how people respond to you during this time of emotional crisis and upheaval.

The most hurtful responses came from those who decided not to get involved. It's important to understand that some people you know very well will not provide any help or comfort. Some of those people could be members of your own family. From the time you begin sharing the news, you may discover the people you hoped to depend on for comfort and support cannot come through for a variety of reasons.

When you experience this letdown, you may be tempted to end those relationships. In the majority of cases, it's a mistake to end relationships based on the lack of support you received during this crisis. If it's still early on your journey, you may not yet have experienced this disappointment and hurt, but you probably will. It's important to understand why this will happen so you don't take it as a personal insult.

Here are the reasons people closest to you could become unavailable or let you down.

> **Cancer is frightening.** Some people are terrified of cancer. Their fear may be a result of previous experiences with a loved one who died. For some people, the images of pain and suffering frighten them away. I believe everyone who knows you will experience this to one degree or another. Your circumstances scare people. You have become a reminder of how frail life truly is. It's extremely frightening to everyone who knows you that you were healthy one day and facing a potentially life-threatening illness the next. As this frightened you, it may frighten other people in your life. Often a response to fear is to flee.

> **Some of your friends and family will be unavailable to you because of a crisis or busyness** in their own lives. They just don't have it within themselves or have the time to be there for you.

> **There are those who would like to help but don't know what to say or do,** so they decide to play it safe and do nothing. In their minds, doing nothing is better than doing something that would add to your pain or suffering.

> **Some will be supportive in the beginning but drop out at some point.** There are different reasons people will drop out. Some get exhausted with how much you might need. Others get exhausted due to the length of time this crisis can last. Still others drop out because they think it's over. Once you've recovered from surgery, especially if you received good news, these folks think your crisis is over. They have no idea how

difficult it is living without a prostate and the many challenges you face after your surgery.

➤ **Some people won't provide support because you expected them to be mind readers**. You may act as if they should have known that receiving the diagnosis of cancer means they should call you. You expected them to reach out to you, so you didn't make any effort to reach out to them. In other words, you didn't receive comfort from these folks because you didn't ask.

➤ **Some won't provide comfort or support because they have not forgiven you for a past offense**. You may or may not have known about this offense. Due to their feelings of anger, bitterness, or unforgiveness, they have no desire to support you in any way.

➤ **You will miss out on support and comfort if it's too difficult or embarrassing for you to share what you are going through**. It's hard to talk about losing urinary control. It may be too personal to share how living without erections is affecting you and your marriage. It's not possible to receive help or comfort when you keep these issues a secret. On the other hand you need to make wise choices regarding the people you share intimate details of your life.

➤ **You will miss out on comfort and support if you withdraw from your spouse.** There may come a time when you feel so ashamed, depressed, anxious, or undeserving of love that you will go into hiding or shut down. I experienced this. When I shut down, I could not give or receive support from my wife. This was a huge loss for both of us.

➤ **You will miss out on comfort if you place all your hope, confidence, and trust only in people**. No one you know is perfect. Therefore, no one person or group can or will meet all your needs. It's my personal belief this disappointment can put you on the path to seek out the only one who is always with you, always available, always wants the best for you, and is able to give you good comfort twenty-four/seven. He's the one who says, "For I know the thoughts that I think toward you, says the LORD, thoughts of peace and not of evil, to give you a future and a hope. Then you will call upon me and go and pray to me, and I will listen to you. And you will seek me and find me, when you search for me with all your heart" (Jeremiah 29:11–14).

To Summarize

There will only be a select few who will be able to stay with you from beginning to end of this crisis. It will be tempting to end your relationships with those who can't provide you with the support you need when you need it. The best advice I can give you is this: do not permanently cut people from your life because they disappointed you. If you do, you will end up lonely and lose important relationships.

Sadly, I had a few relationships that came to an end at different points of my journey. In those relationships, looking back, I can say I didn't realize how broken those relationships were prior to my receiving the diagnosis of prostate cancer. The cancer diagnosis shined a light into the cracks in these relationships. Since there was absolutely no desire to work things out, these relationships ended.

If you experience relationships that end after your diagnosis of cancer, it's highly likely those relationships had areas of hurt, disappointment, or unforgiveness prior to your receiving the diagnosis. These friends or family members might not ever come back into your life. In fact, you may discover they were never there for you to begin with. Whether these people ever come back, I believe my faith calls me to forgive everyone who either disappointed or abandoned me.

That said, the process of reconciling means both parties want to do what it takes to make this happen. You can't heal a relationship by yourself. When someone is closed to the possibility of reconciliation, you need to grieve the loss of that relationship and move on. From the opposite direction, there will be times when it's important to overlook your disappointment with the lack of support and continue with those relationships. I can think of a few people who came, left, and then came back again. They were good friends. There was no way I'd let feelings of disappointment ruin our friendship.

Questions to Consider

1. What expectations for support do you have from your partner?

2. Based on your history, are those expectations realistic?

3. What expectations do you have from your family and friends?

4. Based on your history, are those expectations realistic?

5. Are you prepared to forgive people who disappoint you? If not, why not?

6. Is God's presence offering you comfort? If so, how? If not, might this be your call to find God?

Chapter 11

Choose a Surgeon, Not a Salesman

When I am about to enter a long-term relationship with a physician, bedside manners play an important role in my decision-making process. But when I need surgery, I'm much more concerned with the surgeon's skill and experience; bedside manners take a backseat. It's possible your urologist may be the doctor who performs your prostate surgery. If not, you will receive a referral to see a urologist who performs open or robotic prostate surgery, depending on your personal preference. For a variety of reasons I share later on, I chose robotic surgery.

The outcome of your surgery, meaning whether you regain urinary and sexual function, is partly dependent upon on the skill of your surgeon. In his book *Dr. Patrick Walsh's Guide to Surviving Prostate Cancer,* Dr. Walsh suggests your surgeon should have performed a minimum of three hundred robotic surgeries.

It's possible a surgeon in private practice will not keep statistics regarding the number of his or her patients who regain urinary control and sexual function. Adding to the confusion is the lack of agreement as to what constitutes urinary control. From a patient's perspective, the definition is simple: you won't need to wear pads. A surgeon may define one pad a day as achieving urinary control. With regard to a return of erectile function, a man who has never needed medication to obtain an erection considers a return of erectile function to be brought to the same place. A surgeon may define a return of erectile function (ED) to occur when a man responds to ED medication. Whenever you get into a discussion about these issues, make sure you define clearly what you consider a return of urinary control and sexual function.

You'll want to know who to contact for issues that may arise after surgery, such as questions regarding catheter care, pain control, bladder spasms, and a host of other issues. It's up to you whether you want to go to a treatment center that specializes in prostate surgery. Treatment centers often have support groups as well as penile rehabilitation specialists. They are more likely to keep statistics regarding surgical outcomes.

A major disadvantage to going to a treatment center is the time, distance, and expense involved in getting treated there. You'll need to travel there three to four times for consultations and pre-surgery testing. This could involve missing work, as well as hotel and travel/parking expenses. If you decide to go this route, ask if the treatment center has any special deals with hotels in the area. When my urologist referred me to UCSF, my first reaction was negative. I didn't want to drive the long distance involved or pay for hotel stays. After careful consideration, prayer, and discovering UCSF was a preferred provider, we came to the decision to go there.

I met with Dr. Carole at UCSF for a pre-surgical consultation. He'd performed thousands of robotic surgeries with very good results. There was something that impressed me more than his skill as a surgeon: at no time did he push me to choose surgery as my treatment option. He and his team spent as much time talking about active surveillance as they did about surgery. I was the one who made the decision to have surgery. At no time did I ever feel under any pressure to choose one treatment over another.

Since I had mesh for hernia repairs on both sides of my

abdomen, Dr. Carole informed me it might be necessary to perform open surgery rather than robotic. I had 100 percent confidence in his ability to perform either procedure. I didn't know which surgery I'd had until it was completed. Dr. Carole informed us he'd been able get under the mesh with the robotic arms.

It was time consuming and expensive to make the decision to have surgery at a prostate cancer treatment center, but it was the right decision.

Questions to Consider/ Things to do

1. What qualities are you looking for in your surgeon?

2. What skills and experience do you want your surgeon to have?

3. Would you prefer to travel to a prostate treatment center or have surgery locally?

4. Write a list of questions you want to ask your surgeon before your first consultation.

Chapter 12

Experiencing Disruptive Moments

Gordon MacDonald, in his book *The Life God Blesses,* talks about life's disruptive moments. Disruptive moments are any events that bring about an unwelcome change in our circumstances, health, or well-being. These changes are accompanied by intense suffering. Our lives are turned topsy-turvy against our will. Disruptive moments are not just for a moment; they can involve suffering that will last for years. Receiving the diagnosis of prostate cancer is a disruptive moment. It's a ten on the Richter scale. Once you've received this diagnosis, your life has forever changed.

A few months after surgery, my pastor gave us the opportunity to speak at our church regarding our experiences with our faith and prostate cancer. These are my notes from that talk.

There are eight things I've learned about disruptive moments.

1. **No one is immune**. Everyone will experience many disruptive moments in his or her lifetime.

2. **There is intense suffering** often in one or more of these areas: physically, emotionally, relationally, psychologically, or spiritually.

3. **Your faith will be tested.** It's often difficult for us to understand why our loving heavenly Father would permit an overwhelming amount of pain and suffering into our lives or in the lives of someone we love.

4. **Disruptive moments are game changers.** They will not leave us the way we are. As a result of the suffering, we will get bitter or better. We have the potential to become more loving and compassionate or more selfish, self-centered, and bitter.

5. **Our normal coping mechanisms often fail** because our past experiences and ways of dealing with things are not sufficient to deal with our disruptive moment.

6. **The older you get, the frequency and intensity of disruptive moments increase.**

7. **Children are not immune from experiencing severe and life-changing disruptive moments.** When you were diagnosed with prostate cancer, your children or grandchildren may have experienced that as a disruptive moment.

8. **Facing a disruptive moment without prayer means you will miss some aid, comfort, or blessings from God.** The Bible is very clear on this: "Yet you do not have because you do not ask" (James 4:2).

Some time ago, I questioned what it was that prevented me from going to God in prayer when I've faced disruptive moments. What I discovered was I had a great deal of confusion about what I can and can't say to God in prayer. I believe there is a specific Bible verse that causes this confusion for many people. It certainly did for me: "Rejoice always, pray without ceasing, in everything give thanks; for this is the will of God in Christ Jesus for you" (1 Thessalonians 5:16–18).

Whenever we are hurting or suffering deeply, we

may feel an intense anger toward God for allowing this pain and suffering to occur. There's probably not an iota of thanksgiving either. Therefore, if you believe "ACTS" (adoration, confession, thanksgiving, and supplication) is the only model for prayer, your anger and lack of gratitude will keep you from praying.

I have great news for you! The Bible teaches us there's more than one way to pray. I've studied the prayers of people in their disruptive moments, and I've learned you can pray to God straight from the heart and don't have to feel adoration or thanksgiving in order to pray. If there is only one thing you take away from this discussion, make it this: *In your disruptive moment, cry out to God in pain and with whatever is in your heart. God will respond to your prayers.* I believe the biggest tragedy that can occur in a disruptive moment isn't about the pain of that moment; the bigger tragedy occurs if you stay away from prayer and miss out on blessings, comfort, help, and spiritual growth God intends for you to experience.

In the last two disruptive moments in my life, I've also learned there are some specific things we can pray for that will be enormously helpful. I knew I needed wisdom, and the Bible gives us this promise in James 1:5–8: "If any of you lacks wisdom, let him ask of God, who gives to all liberally and without reproach, and it will be given to him." Facing a disruptive moment without God's wisdom is a foolish thing to do.

In a previous season of illness, I learned how easy it was to lose my sense of humor and just how important laughter is. Proverbs 17:22 says, "A merry heart does good, like medicine." I prayed we would find humor and things to laugh about. God was gracious and answered this prayer as well. Shortly after I was diagnosed, we went out to dinner with a couple from our church. All of us expected it to be a subdued or depressing dinner. What happened is, we found something cancer-related that was uproariously funny. Our night out was filled with laughter. It was an amazing evening and a gift from God. Just recently a friend sent me a book by Dr. Seuss titled *You're Only Old Once! A Book for Obsolete Children*. This is a very funny book!

I prayed for comfort: "Praise be to the God and Father of our Lord Jesus Christ, the Father of compassion and the God of all comfort, who comforts us in all our troubles, so that we can comfort those in any trouble with the comfort we ourselves have received from God" (2 Corinthians 1:3–4).

Sometimes God's comfort is easy to recognize because our sorrow is turned into joy: "You have turned for me my mourning into dancing; You have put off my sackcloth and clothed me with gladness" (Psalm 30:11).

That's my favorite way to experience God's comfort. However, there are some disruptive moments that bring pain to our hearts and tears to our eyes for as long as we live. God comforts us when we have that kind of pain as well, but it's easy to miss because the sorrow remains with us. So what does God's comfort look like in the midst of pain and sorrow that will not go away? And where can that comfort be found? Here's where I need to go to the Bible and camp out with God's promises.

The promises I found may not be the promises you'll need, but I'll share two of God's promises that bring comfort to my heart and to my soul: "And not only that, but we also glory in tribulations, knowing that tribulation produces perseverance; and perseverance, character; and character, hope" (Romans 5:3).

This verse reminds me there are certain character traits God wants to build into my life, and they are learned on the path of suffering. To know God is working in my disruptive moments to give me character traits that I need in this life and will also be enjoyed throughout eternity brings me great comfort. Another important verse to me is, "For I know the thoughts that I think toward you, says the LORD, thoughts of peace and not of evil, to give you a future and a hope" (Jeremiah 29:11).

This verse reminds me to trust God's good intentions

and love in the midst of painful or difficult circumstances. I'm always comforted when I'm reminded we have an eternal home where God wipes away every tear from our eyes, a home where there will be no more death, sorrow, crying, or pain. It's a world in which we have our citizenship and where we will spend eternity.

There are many wonderful promises in the Bible, and it's good to be anchored to some of these promises before a storm comes, because your faith will be tested. Something else was made quite clear to us: we could not face my diagnosis of cancer alone.

As Jesus prayed before He chose His disciples, we need to pray that God would bring the right people to us and we'd have wisdom to know who to put on our team. We realized we needed a team of people to help us with:

1. Prayer

2. Spiritual support

3. Emotional support

4. Information about prostate cancer

5. Answering medical questions (and we would need a team we could trust)

6. We needed people who would speak truth into our lives and who knew our strengths and weaknesses.

I also found a great need for people on my team who had traveled farther along the road I was traveling. A biblical example of this is Mary going to her cousin Elizabeth because she was further along the path of a miraculous birth and was probably the only person on the planet divinely prepared to believe and support Mary. Mary stayed with Elizabeth for three months.

Through every phase of my illness, I needed to hear from men who'd traveled further along the path I was traveling. To do this, I joined two online prostate cancer support groups. From these groups I've been blessed with comfort and valuable information that's been useful to me in every phase of this illness. Once you have your team together, pray for them!

In every disruptive moment of my life, I've always been pleasantly surprised by acts of kindness. Some examples to look for:

♦ An invitation for coffee or a meal out

♦ Cards

♦ Phone calls

♦ E-mails

♦ Words of wisdom and support

♦ Gifts (like a copy of this book)

Whenever any of these events occurred, I considered it a blessing. From the opposite direction, there's always been at least one major disappointment. This time, that came from a friend I've known for more than half my life. I thought he would stay with me closer than a brother. Sadly, weeks and sometimes a month would go by before we would speak, and if I wanted to talk with him, I'd be the one to reach out. I found it difficult to understand why he was out of touch for long periods of time when I needed his friendship and support.

This experience taught me a valuable lesson. I learned not to kick people out of my life because they disappointed me in a disruptive moment. This lesson is found in the Bible as well. Jesus experienced disappointment and abandonment when His team of disciples fell asleep in the garden in Jesus' moment of great need. After He was arrested, they all ran away. Peter went so far as to deny he ever knew Jesus. Despite disappointment and abandonment, Jesus didn't kick His disciples off His team.

So don't expect everyone on your team to meet your expectations all the time, and don't kick people out of your life for a single disappointment. If you've kicked someone out of your life, tell him or her you were convicted at church of doing something wrong, and invite that person back into your life. You can do what I do. I just tell him or her, "I've acted like a jerk and I'd like you back in my life." Sadly (or happily), no one has ever disagreed with me. We both agree I'm a jerk, and the friendship is restored.

Almost everything I've said today can be summarized with a single eight-word Bible verse: "Is anyone among you suffering? Let him pray" (James 5:13).

I have shared some specific things to pray for in disruptive moments and a testimony that God will answer your prayers—not necessarily in ways you want but in ways you need. Remember, we were not designed to go through disruptive moments alone. Sometimes it's pain and sometimes it's shame that keeps us from reaching out, but we need a team.

Disruptive moments involve suffering. If you decide to face your disruptive moments alone, you will add additional and unnecessary suffering and pain to you and to those you love the most in the world. As you face all the disruptive moments prostate surgery brings to your life, rely on your team, rely on prayer, and rely on the Lord. If Jesus took the time to put together a team for His earthly ministry, why would you consider going through this illness alone?

Putting together a team isn't an easy task. It takes time to find the right people. It involves searching. It involves taking the risk of telling people what's really going on in your life. Not everyone you'd like on your team will agree to join. Almost everyone will disappoint you at one time or another. In addition, some team members will drift in and out. You may find, as I did, that it's necessary to remove people, and it's a lot of work to keep a team together. That's why there will be times when it feels as if having a team is more trouble than it's worth.

There's something else that's important for a couple to realize. While you might find people who are on both your teams, each of you may have different team members as well. There's nothing wrong with that, but there is one potential danger. If you are married, I advise you not to choose a member of the opposite sex to provide you with emotional support. There is a danger of having an emotional or physical affair, or both.

You might be thinking, *With the hassles, disappointments, and potential hurt, why on earth would I want to put together a team?* I want to assure you that putting together a team is the right thing to do. In fact, the Bible tells us this: "Two are better than one, because they have a good reward for their labor. For if they fall, one will lift up his companion. But woe to him who is alone when he falls, for he has no one to help him up. Again, if two lie down together, they will keep warm; but how can one be warm alone? Though one may be overpowered by another, two can withstand him. And a threefold cord is not quickly broken" (Ecclesiastes 4:9–12).

So choose your team wisely, carefully, and prayerfully.

Questions to Consider

1. What people come to mind as people you'd like on your team?

2. Do you know any men who've had prostate cancer you might talk to?

3. Would you feel more comfortable with a face-to-face support group, or would you prefer an Internet support group?

4. Is there someone you'd like to pray for you? Will you call him or her?

5. Do you think it's important for you to pray? If so, will you begin to do this?

Chapter 13

Checking in so You Don't Check Out

Once Churchill and Lady Astor were
discussing the role of women in Parliament,
a subject she strongly believed in and
Churchill opposed. Somewhat frustrated
with the conversation, Lady Astor said in
exasperation, "Sir Winston, if I were your
wife I'd put arsenic in your coffee." To
which Churchill replied, "Madam, if I were
your husband, I'd drink it."

—Allen Klein, *Healing Power of Humor*

The diagnosis of prostate cancer will affect you and your
marriage for the rest of your life. The only question is,
will you end up closer to your spouse, with your marriage
strengthened, or will you end up unhappy, angry, frustrated,
more distant from each other, or divorced? You might
wonder why I am mentioning this now. You are already
under enough stress. You have too much on your plate to
worry about the state of your marriage.

When I'm about to take a long journey in my car, I
usually make sure I'm up to date on all my scheduled

maintenance. If I'm due for an oil change, tire rotation, or anything else, I'll get it all done. I want to make sure my car is ready for the long journey. I do all this to minimize my chances of getting stuck alongside the road. My goal is to arrive at my destination without a preventable breakdown.

What's true about cars is also true about marriages. The state of your marriage at this moment in time depends upon how well you've met each other's emotional needs. If one or both of you are chronically dissatisfied or unhappy, your relationship is in need of extensive repairs. My advice is to do the same thing for your marriage as you would for your car. Now is a good time to schedule a "tune-up and preventive maintenance" for your relationship. You are heading for a long and difficult journey together.

Most men reading this will find themselves resisting what I'm advising here. In his book *Seven Principles for Making Marriage Work* John Gottman found that more than 80 percent of the time, it's the wife who brings up sticky marital issues while the husband tries to avoid discussing them. This isn't a symptom of a troubled marriage; it's true in most happy marriages as well.

Therefore, it's likely the overwhelming majority of men will find excuses to skip this task. As someone who has walked further along this road than you have, I can say with a voice of experience that as tough as it is for you now, it's possible it can and will get worse after surgery. If you choose to skip the marital tune-up, you may find yourself isolated while you cope with the most stressful and painful emotions you've ever experienced in your life.

Men, listen up. If you want to ignore this task, you are putting yourself and your marriage at risk. In a relatively short time after surgery, you may find yourself hating the quality of your life so much you will regret your choice to treat your cancer. In fact, you could end up so depressed you won't enjoy your life even if surgery cures your cancer. I cannot even put into words how important it is to have your wife's love, comfort, and support. From the other direction, your wife needs you to hear her struggles as well. She will need your comfort and support as much as you need hers. You are on an extremely stressful journey. God designed marriage so you would have a helpmate to share both the pleasures and pain that life brings. When you were married, you promised to stay together in sickness and in health. This may be the first time in your marriage or relationship where you are facing a sickness that involves a life-threatening disease.

I received a comment on my online diary from a man recently diagnosed with prostate cancer. He wrote, "My emotions are all over the place. I'm withdrawing from social things ... arguing with my wife ... avoiding any kind of intimacy." This is not an unusual remark. It's typical, so make and take time to straighten out your marriage now. At this point in the journey, you may spend much of your free time worrying or zoning out by the TV or with a favorite hobby. Borrow some of that time and make it a top priority to prepare your marriage for the storms ahead.

There are some couples who are starting this journey with marriages that are already troubled. If one or both of you agree to many of the statements made below, I would advise you to skip the exercises in this chapter and seek professional help to strengthen your marriage. It's up to the members of each couple to decide whether they have the skills necessary to tune up their marriage. I want to give you some indications of when it would be wise to seek out professional help to strengthen your marriage for storms ahead. Please put a checkmark in the statements that *currently* are true about your relationship:

- ❏ Defensiveness—one or both of you are quick to get angry or blame the other when in conflict.

- ❏ You frequently think you'd be better off alone than together.

❑ Your communication is marked by hostility or criticism.

❑ You are highly dissatisfied with the state of your emotional connection to one another.

❑ You are highly dissatisfied with your sexual relationship.

❑ You believe you need professional help, but the other refuses to go.

❑ You blame your spouse for your unhappiness. You think he or she is the only one who needs to change.

❑ There is a loss of goodwill between you. When you've lost your goodwill toward your partner, almost everything he or she does will be seen in a negative light. From the other direction, anything positive is ignored, unnoticed, or forgotten.

❑ You have an unforgiving spirit. You keep careful records of the wrongdoings of your partner and bring them up continually, either in your mind or to your partner.

❑ There is an inability to hear one another accurately. Because of unresolved issues, you can't hear what's going on in the present. Instead you might end up fighting about old unresolved conflicts. From the other direction, one partner will shut down and refuse to listen or deal with the issue.

❑ When you resolve conflicts, your primary goal is get your way or win at all costs.

❑ When you resolve conflicts, your partner becomes your enemy rather than the problem that was dividing you.

❑ Conflicts end with one or both of you feeling worse about your relationship.

If you've placed a check in three or more of these

boxes, it's likely many of the behaviors listed below will prevent you from resolving your marital conflicts on your own. These are behaviors that escalate rather than resolve conflict:

- ☐ Yelling
- ☐ Lying
- ☐ Blaming
- ☐ Sarcasm
- ☐ Criticism
- ☐ Leaving the room or your house
- ☐ The silent treatment; this can go on for hours, days, weeks, or months.
- ☐ Withholding sex
- ☐ Hostile humor
- ☐ Cross-complaining
- ☐ Interrupting
- ☐ Exaggerating
- ☐ Character attacks
- ☐ Put downs
- ☐ Aggressive use of touch
- ☐ Hostile use of humor
- ☐ Threats of physical violence

Look back and review how many boxes were checked off on both lists. The more boxes that were checked, the more difficult it will be for you to tune up your marriage without professional help. If you are having surgery at a major treatment center, it is possible they have counseling services. Take advantage of that opportunity.

Earlier in our marriage, Brenda and I were unable to break up repetitive and destructive fights with each other. My wife was the first to recognize we needed help. Like most men, I foolishly disagreed. Brenda said if I continued to refuse to get help for our marriage, we'd need to remodel our garage. When I asked why, she said it was because the garage would become my bedroom. That was where I was going to live until I agreed to get help, and then she told me to choose.

I was so ticked off I said, "I'll think about it and get back to you." My decision to get help for our marriage was one of the best decisions I've made. We also started a group at our church called "Committed Couples." A group of us met for more than a decade, growing our marriages and sharing our lives and struggles together.

There's no doubt in my mind Brenda and I would have divorced years ago if we had not taken those steps to help our marriage. Now is not the time to act foolishly. If one of you believe your relationship needs help, both of you should agree to seek that help. Violent storms are on the horizon. It's my belief if one of you says, "We need help," and the other refuses, your relationship needs more help than you can possibly know. In fact, the words of the robot from the TV show *Lost in Space* comes to mind: "Danger, Will Robinson."

I don't know anyone who would refuse to take his car to a mechanic for a repair if the tires were bald, the spark plugs were misfiring, or the check engine light came on. Yet I've seen many marriages end in divorce because of a stubborn refusal to get help when things were going poorly in the relationship. Why are men more willing to do what's necessary to take care of their cars than they are to help their marriage? I suspect it has to do with the fact most men lack the skills and seek to avoid dealing with emotional issues. For this reason I highly recommend that *every* couple read *The Seven Principles for Making Marriage Work* by Gottman and Silver. If one of you refuse, the other can read it alone. There's an excellent chance you will learn some skills that can move your relationship in a positive direction.

Men, listen up: if one or both of you are chronically

unhappy, isolated, and angry or disappointed, your marriage will end up causing additional stress to both of you rather than becoming a safe harbor in a storm. Deciding you need help in your marriage now is as wise as taking care of your car when it's in obvious need of repair. Treat your marriage with at least the same care you give your car.

Finding the right help takes time. Not every counselor is competent. If you have a religious affiliation, your church, temple, or mosque may provide counseling services or know someone to refer. There are also a number of online services to help you locate a therapist in your area. Use your favorite search engine, and type in "how to find a therapist for marital counseling." Another great resource is friends or family who may know of a good therapist in your area.

What's true about prostate cancer is also true about healing your marriage. The first step is admitting something is wrong. Without taking that step, there will be no movement toward healing. It's possible this awful experience with prostate cancer can bring you closer together than you've ever been. This will not happen naturally; it will take diligent work and intentionality. If you ignore your relationship by deciding to roll the dice and let things land as they may, the odds are you will end up distant from one another and very unhappy. I hope you are wise enough to work on your relationship.

Just as there are some car problems you can fix yourself, there are many couples who can perform a marital tune-up without outside help. Here are some indicators to suggest you can perform a marital tune-up as a couple:

❏ Overall you have a feeling of goodwill toward your spouse and your marriage.

❏ You have a history of successfully sharing difficult or painful emotions.

❏ You can listen to each other without interrupting or getting defensive.

❏ You value listening to each other more than fixing one another.

❏ You have a forgiving spirit.

❏ You have friends who can speak truth into your life.

When you search for information at a library or online, you don't get angry or defensive. You look for that information with a curious and inquisitive spirit. That's the spirit you'll need as you answer the survey questions below.

As you discuss the areas where you need work or are dissatisfied, rather than complaining of behaviors you don't like, attempt to describe a positive behavior you'd like. For example, let's say a wife is bringing up an important topic while the husband is watching TV. The wife's complaint would sound like this: "You never listen to me." A positive request would sound like this: "I'd like to find a time without distractions when we can discuss things that are important to me."

If you begin a discussion and either of you become angry or defensive, stop discussing the topic. Find out what is fueling your defensive attitude, and deal with this first before you attempt to resolve a conflict. There are some conflicts you may not have the skills to resolve alone. You may need to call in a trusted friend, a pastor, or a therapist to help you.

Here are some areas in your relationship
to evaluate and discuss together:

List of Behaviors	Very Satisfied	Satisfied	Needs Work	Dissatisfied	Very Dissatisfied
Physical touch					
Time spent having fun					
Our emotional connection					
Encouraging each other					
How decisions are made					
How we resolve conflicts together					
Our spiritual connection					
How we deal with our children together					
How we manage money					
How we deal with relatives					
What we think of the friends we have					

	Very Satisfied	Satisfied	Needs Work	Dissatisfied	Very Dissatisfied
The romance in our lives					
Our foreplay					
The frequency of sex					
Satisfaction from sex					
Helpful Communication Styles					
Actively listen					
Reflect back what you've heard					
Enjoyable use of humor					
Praise/compliment each other					
Encourage each other					
Take responsibility for behavior					
Able to admit when you are wrong					
Have emotional self-control					

	Very Satisfied	Satisfied	Needs Work	Dissatisfied	Very Dissatisfied
Use positive nonverbal behavior					
Accept partner's feelings					
Express sorrow for wrongdoing					
Demonstrate a willingness to change					
Tender use of physical touch					
Speak the truth in love					
Make positive assumptions about partner					
Use effective problem solving					
Hurtful Styles of Communication					
Blames the other for most problems					
Uses sarcasm					
Often critical of partner					

Uses verbal or physical threats				
Storms out of the house				
Uses the silent treatment				
Withholds sex				
Uses hostile humor				
Interrupting				
Cross-complaining				
Put downs				
Aggressive use of touch				
Attacks the character of his or her partner				
Uses negative nonverbal behavior				
Withdraws or ignores partner				

Questions to Discuss after the Survey Is Completed

1. What are the positive things you notice about your relationship? Take time to compliment one another for those areas.

2. What did you learn about the way you communicate?

3. What strengths do you have that make it easy to speak with you?

4. What areas of weakness do you have that make it difficult to speak with you?

5. What family member or friend do you resemble the most?

6. Is this who you want to imitate? If so, why, and if not, why not?

7. What styles of communication do you have that strengthen your marriage?

8. What styles of communication are present that hurt your marriage?

9. Were there any surprises in areas that need work? What were they?

10. Did any of your partner's answers hurt you in any way? Discuss this with each other.

11. Agree to find ways to discuss those areas that need work so you can strengthen your marriage.

12. Which areas will be easy to change? Which present more difficulty and why?

13. Are there areas you refuse to change? How will your refusal affect your marriage?

14. Are there areas you will not be able to change without seeking outside help? If so, will you do that?

There are a number of things you can do on your own to make positive changes in your marriage. One of those boils down to a simple mathematical formula, which John Gottman, in his book *Why Marriages Succeed or Fail,* discovered. In healthy marriages, where couples maintain goodwill toward one another, they must have a five-to-one ratio of positive interactions to negative interaction. When that ratio is lower, the level of dissatisfaction in marriage increases.

An important change to make if you are dissatisfied or unhappy in your marriage is to achieve this five-to-one ratio. Here are some suggestions to help you do this.

❒ How you greet and separate from one another gives some indication about your feelings toward one another, so pay attention to this. In the morning when you first wake up, start your day by sharing a kind word and some form of positive physical touch, such as a hug or a kiss. Plan to do this again when you see each other before and after work. Take the time to greet and separate from each other warmly. To help you get in the spirit of this idea, think back to the days when it was difficult or painful to say good-bye. Try to regain some of those feelings, and use them to show positive regard and positive physical touch before heading out the door to mow the lawn or run an errand. Take time to do more than grunt, "Doing the lawn now." Find a way to spend a few moments with each other to make your leaving memorable and meaningful to each other. A kind word of affection, a hug, a kiss—whatever you agree to, do it.

❐ Make an effort and search diligently to find ways to say something nice or complimentary and express positive affection with words and physical touch multiple times a day. Do this as if your marriage depends on it because there's a good chance it does.

❐ Place a guard on your tongue. The function of a guard is make sure someone or something is protected. In other words, it's the guard who determines who and what comes in or goes out. Here are some things the guard of your tongue must prevent from escaping: character assassinations, which often start out with, "You always are_____ (late, sloppy, irresponsible, etc.)"; hostile humor; unkind words; and criticism.

❐ Find time for mutually enjoyable activities.

❐ Make time to connect with each other emotionally. Take a minimum of ten to twenty minutes every day and ask:

1. How are you doing today?

2. What's bothering you the most?

3. What things bring joy or peace into your life?

4. What things brought distress into your life?

Take a look at how you both filled out your questionnaire, and discuss the following:

♦ Notice the things you do well together. Take time to compliment each other about how well you each do things.

♦ Notice the things you need to work on. Each of

you take turns giving a vision of how you'd like those areas to improve. In other words, talk about what behaviors you need to change in order to reach your vision.

♦ If you are able, take a fun and/or romantic trip for a few days during the weeks while you are waiting for surgery or other treatment options.

I hope you take this chapter seriously because even the best of marriages will find this journey extremely stressful.

You need good communication styles and goodwill toward each other in order to help one another cope with the highly stressful journey you both are on. Without goodwill and effective communication skills, it's highly likely the diagnosis of cancer and coping with the aftermath of surgery will result in your feeling emotionally disconnected from one another.

If you have a long history of highly satisfying sex together, this part of your relationship may suffer for years to come. It's essential to take the time to prepare your marriage for the hazardous journey ahead.

If your sense of discouragement is so high right now that you've lost your desire or hope for a better marriage, it's an important indication that you need to get outside help. I hope you won't let your relationship history, discouragement, stubbornness, or shame, stop you from seeking help.

Right now one or both of you may be stuck in negativity, but it is possible to heal your marriage. I encourage you to do this and take this task as seriously as finding the right treatment option for your prostate cancer.

Things to Do to Help Your Relationship

♦ Tell your partner three or four things he or she can do on a regular basis that you'll appreciate.

Make sure you thank your partner each and every time he or she does those things.

♦ Find ways to bring your conversations to a 5:1 ratio, where positive things are said five times more than negative things.

♦ Identify some activities you both find enjoyable and spend time doing those things together.

♦ Compliment each other a minimum of twice a day.

♦ Affectionately touch each other for the sake of enjoying touch rather than limit the use of touching as a signal you are interested in sex. In other words, enjoy holding hands, back rubs, and other forms of touch to bring both of you pleasure.

♦ If you have a history of positive sexual experiences use this time to create many more positive memories.

♦ If your sex life is filled with conflict or has a long history of disappointment, that's often a symptom there are many other issues than need to be resolved. Make a plan to work together or with a professional to get the help you need to make your relationship emotionally and physically more satisfying for both of you.

Chapter 14

Why I Chose Surgery

Receiving the diagnosis of prostate cancer was the most frightening experience I'd ever faced. There were so many different treatment options to choose from. Each of those options had certain advantages and each had potentially serious downsides.

Choosing active surveillance, means you will monitor your cancer until tests show the cancer is progressing. Some men are able to go decades without aggressive treatment. The only easy decision was to rule out active surveillance. My PSA doubled in fewer than eight months, and I had a palpable lump. I was certain I needed to treat my prostate cancer.

My first impulse was to choose the treatment that would be most convenient. I didn't want to miss any time from work. I didn't want to drive long distances. I didn't want to have to come back multiple times for treatment, as you need to do with radiation. The only treatment option that met all my initial criteria was brachytherapy, often referred to as "seeds. This form of treatment involves the placement of radioactive seeds inside the prostate gland. In the early stages of decision making, when convenience was my top priority, seed implantation was my first choice.

Sometime later I added two more criteria into the decision-making process. I wanted to know about fifteen-year survival rates and potentially life-altering side effects. I learned that men with my urological history tend to do poorly with seed implantation. I visited a few online support groups and found men who suffered lifelong rectal and urinary troubles. The most severe case was a man who required a permanent catheter. If there was a one in a thousand chance I'd need a permanent catheter, the risk would be too high.

At that point, convenience was taken off my list of priorities. My top priority became fifteen-year survival rates. After that came the quality-of-life issues. I decided surgery offered me the best long-term survival rates. Currently, robotic surgery is heavily marketed to men with prostate cancer. Hospitals and treatment centers have spent more than a million dollars to purchase their robotic equipment. It seems every treatment center and urological practice that performs robotic surgery is involved with marketing this procedure to men with prostate cancer.

Since I did the majority of my research on the web, I fell hook, line, and sinker for all the misleading claims that are made online regarding robotic surgery. Promises of a one-day hospital stay and rapid return of both urinary and sexual function sounded great to me.

Looking back, I really can't determine how much the marketing campaigns I read and listened to in cyberspace affected my decision to have surgery. I believed everything I read. I went into surgery expecting my post-surgical life was going to be a cakewalk. I believe the majority of men who choose surgery will be bitterly disappointed if your expectations about post-surgical life come from men who are cherry-picked for promotional advertising.

There were additional reasons I chose surgery that had nothing to do with marketing. I wanted the treatment option that could remove 100 percent of the prostate cancer cells from my body. Surgery was the only treatment option that could give me the peace of mind I needed. I knew I could not and would not experience a single day of peace if I had to live with the idea that cancer cells were still alive and well in my prostate, working twenty-four/seven to escape my prostate with the goal of killing me. The fact that this process could take fifteen years gave me zero comfort. My personality and fears were important factors I had to take into consideration. Brenda felt the same way.

In addition, I've experienced a long history of prostate issues as a result of BPH (benign prostatic hypertrophy, or an enlarged prostate). I had not slept through the night in more than a decade due to a frequent need to urinate. Waking up two to three times a night became an everyday occurrence. Years ago I had surgery to improve my urine flow. Unfortunately, the difficulty returned. My urologist was putting off a second surgery by using medication for as long as possible. Prior to the diagnosis of prostate cancer, my urine flow was getting progressively worse. I knew it was only of matter of time before I'd need another surgical procedure on my prostate.

There were cancer-related considerations as well. I had a palpable lump. My PSA came close to doubling in eight months. I expected to live another fifteen years, and I was healthy enough for surgery. The idea of getting rid of my prostate appealed to me. Prior to my diagnosis of prostate cancer, I thought of my prostate as a pesky organ that was interfering with the quality of my life to a greater degree with every passing year. Now that cancer cells resided there, I thought this was the right time for my prostate and me to go our separate ways. Those were the reasons I came to the decision to leave my prostate in San Francisco.

Questions/Thoughts to Consider

1. How has reading about my experiences influenced your attitude about surgery? (Come back to this question after reading the entire book)

2. If you decide on surgery, what things can you do to prepare yourself for challenges and issues surgery will bring into your life as well as into your relationships?

3. Are there any questions you'd like answered before making a decision?

4. Do you have a team in place to support you after surgery?

5. How you will continue to love one another during the time you may lose both urinary control and erectile function?

6. What things would you like to do individually and as a couple before you have surgery?

Chapter 15

In or out of Network—A Ten Thousand Dollar Question

If you belong to an HMO, you can skip this chapter. If you have a PPO, which allows you to choose treatment centers, skipping this chapter could cost you thousands of dollars, so read this chapter carefully. After that, make the phone calls necessary to protect your hard-earned money.

My local urologist wanted me to go to UCSF for surgery. Since I had PPO coverage, I could have my treatment anywhere that accepted my insurance. There is a very important catch. When your doctor makes a referral to a treatment center and that center accepts your insurance, it does not mean that treatment center is a preferred provider.

Most PPOs limit their out-of-network payments to the "reasonable and customary charges for services provided." Hearing this may give you a false sense of security. You might assume out-of-network service providers accept the dollar amounts your insurance company deems reasonable and customary. In the majority of cases, they won't. If you do not learn whether your treatment center or surgeon is a preferred provider, a few months after surgery you could discover you are personally liable to pay tens of thousands of dollars your insurance company doesn't cover.

I don't know your financial resources, but I know mine. I couldn't afford for that to happen. Therefore, before I accepted my urologist's referral, it was necessary to find out if UCSF was an in-network or out-of-network provider. I thought this would be an easy task. It wasn't.

I began by calling my health insurance company's customer service line. I asked a very simple question. I asked if UCSF was a preferred network provider. They confirmed that UCSF was a preferred provider, but they gave me a warning. They told me their list was thirty days old. Therefore, it was possible to go into the hospital, get the bill, and discover they are no longer in-network providers. They told me the only way to get current information was to contact my treatment center.

So I called UCSF. I'm not sure which department I was transferred to. I gave them my insurance information and asked if they were an in-network provider. After placing me on hold for a long time, they came back on the line and told me to contact my insurance company! Obviously that was the wrong answer, so I asked to be transferred to admitting. They told me that after I was discharged, I could find out what my insurance covered and didn't cover. I wasn't about to risk losing a good deal of my life's savings because I couldn't get a clear answer. I hung up and took a few minutes to calm down. I made another call to UCSF and asked for the department that handled the billing. I told them I needed to know if they were an approved provider for my insurance company.

They told me they were. Relief! I could receive treatment at UCSF. Unfortunately, that didn't end my problem. Each doctor and each lab could be either in-network or out-of-network. I decided this was too much work, so I made one additional call to my surgeon's office to make sure he was an in-network provider. Once I found out he was, I was willing to stop there and take my chances with the rest of the providers.

Your urologist will refer you to a surgeon and a treatment

center. Once they have your insurance information and agree to see you, you cannot assume the treatment center or your surgeon is a preferred provider. You need to call and confirm this with your surgeon and treatment center. If you can't afford to owe thousands of dollars in out-of-pocket costs for your treatment, take the time to call your surgeon's office and the billing department of your treatment center. Make sure they are in-network providers for your insurance company. This is also true if your doctor ordered a bone scan. Verify the facility performing the scan is in network. If you don't, you could end up owing that facility thousands of dollars.

If you have an HSA (health savings account), there is another way you can save some money. If you have any out of pocket expenses for your medical care, you may use the funds from HSA to pay for your medical expenses not covered by your insurance. Another way you can save money is to obtain a prescription from your urologist or surgeon for diapers and pads. This will enable to you use your HSA to purchase these items.

Chapter 16

The Longest Wait
of Your Life

The time between your biopsy and your surgery will be a minimum of four to six weeks. This wait is necessary. Your rectum was punctured during the biopsy and needs to heal completely before your surgery. The question and challenge presented to every man is how you will use your time between your biopsy and your surgery. Sadly, I must confess I used this time poorly for a number of reasons. I am going to share the mistakes I made in the hope you can learn from them and use this precious time differently.

The trauma of receiving the diagnosis of prostate cancer was extremely stressful and terrifying emotionally. Like many men who receive this diagnosis in their fifties, I had to go to work, keep my emotions under control, and carry out my day-to-day responsibilities. Even though I chose surgery, I still spent time trying to absorb a lot of information in order to understand my biopsy results and prepare for surgery. If you are in a relationship and have children or extended family and friends, you need to decide what you will share with those people in your life, including your employer and co-workers.

There were several worries that prevented me from using my time wisely while I was waiting for surgery. After

I experienced urinary difficulty after my bone scan and temporary impotence after my biopsy, I became convinced this was only the beginning of my experiencing issues outside the statistical norms. This conclusion was an additional burden to cope with. Right or wrong, since the biopsy affected my ability to have an erection for two weeks, I began to worry I could be one of those men who would not regain their erectile abilities after surgery. My level of anxiety and fear were off the charts.

When Brenda and I discussed the possibility of my taking some time off from work just to get away and have a good time, I didn't think I was capable of letting things go or having a good time. I posted my dilemma on a support forum. I titled my thread, "To Go away or Not to Go Away—That's the Question." A man who'd already had surgery gave me the following advice: "Don't bother traveling or taking a vacation because you won't enjoy it." He advised me to wait until after surgery. His advice made perfect sense to me, so I followed it. To this day, I seriously regret following that advice.

If you and your spouse can afford to take time off from work and go someplace special, do it. Make sure it's a place you both can have a fun-filled, wonderful time together. If you have an enjoyable sex life together, make sure you take time for romance as well. After surgery you may not have a spontaneous erection again for eighteen to twenty-four months. It's also possible you'll have a complete loss of urinary control for months. Last but not least, the pleasurable sensation of ejaculation is lost forever following surgery. These are your last weeks when everything in your body is working the way it's supposed to work. Emotionally you may feel like I did—too shell-shocked to enjoy anything. Looking back, I wish I'd taken the time to get away and create special memories. I wish I could say I made good use of the time I spent waiting for surgery. The sad fact is, I didn't. There are destructive and constructive ways to cope with the diagnosis of cancer and your pre-surgery anxiety.

Destructive things to do:

- ❖ Isolate yourself from the people who love you.
- ❖ Use drugs or alcohol to alter your mood.
- ❖ Become more selfish. Decide to live as if your life is the only one that matters.
- ❖ Obsessively worry day and night.
- ❖ Lose sleep.

Constructive things to do:

- ◆ Get away. Go on vacation or stay at home taking time to have fun.
- ◆ Enjoy romantic times together.
- ◆ Find ways to express your love to friends and family.
- ◆ Do what's in your power to do to heal any fractured relationships.
- ◆ Pray together, and have people praying for you and your partner.
- ◆ Check out our pre-surgery forum at whereisyourprostate.com.

I hope you can learn from my mistakes and use this time between surgery in ways that will create positive experiences and memories with those you love. Ask yourself, "Will I wait wisely?"

Chapter 17

Things to Know and Do Before and After Surgery

Based on my experiences, here are some things to deal with prior to your surgery. I neglected to discuss the issue of post-surgical pain control with my doctor prior to surgery. I wrongly assumed my post-surgical pain would be adequately managed. I spent the first night in the hospital sleepless and in a significant amount of pain. I was provided with injections for pain every few hours. I found this was an ineffective way to manage my pain the first night following surgery. I believe every man who is about to have his prostate removed should be given the option for pain control that Dr. Walsh offers at Johns Hopkins. It's called patient-controlled analgesia (PCA). PCA is a computerized pump that safely permits you to push a button and deliver small amounts of pain medicine into your IV line, usually in your arm. If I had to do it over again, I'd ask for PCA. Johns Hopkins offers this type of pain control for the first night post-surgery. The next day you are given pain pills. By my second night, pain pills effectively managed my pain.

You can't expect pain medication to provide you with a 100 percent relief of pain and discomfort following surgery. That's not going to happen. However, your pain level should be managed well. In other words, if you think of pain on a scale of zero to ten, with ten being the highest level, you are not receiving appropriate pain management if your pain is in the seven-to-ten range. If your pain is somewhere between three and five, that may be the best it's going to get. Don't expect to be medicated down to zero.

From the opposite direction, if your post-surgical pain level is between seven and ten, it's important for you to inform the hospital staff and/or your surgeon so an adjustment can be made. I wish I had discussed an alternative method of pain control be put into my chart prior to surgery so I could have switched methods sometime during that first night. I was in serious pain following surgery, and the medication I was prescribed did little to ease it.

There are a number of sources of pain or discomfort you may experience following surgery. Discuss these issues with your surgeon so orders are in your chart:

✓ **Bladder spasms** are painful contractions of the bladder, which often begins once your catheter is inserted. Some men never have a single bladder spasm. I was in a small group of men who continued to have painful bladder spasms many months following after my catheter was pulled. Bladder spasm pain can be mild or severe. My pain was severe. Thankfully, there are effective medications available to relieve painful bladder spasms.

✓ **Catheter irritation**. The tip of your penis could become irritated from the catheter. I found topical analgesic Lidocaine helped make the pain tolerable.

✓ **Nausea/vomiting**. Speak with your anesthesiologist about receiving medication for nausea during surgery. Because I did this, I did not throw up in the recovery room. Unfortunately, I made the mistake of not asking my surgeon for anti-nausea medication after surgery. Because of this mistake, I threw up my breakfast the following morning. Vomiting caused me extreme pain in my abdomen. After that experience, I asked my surgeon for anti-nausea medication and kept my food down. With the amount of pain involved with post-surgical vomiting, it's better to be safe than sorry.

✓ **Sleeplessness**. Due to pain, noise, or other reasons, you may, like me, be unable to get significant or consecutive hours of sleep. My suggestion is to ask your surgeon for medication to help you sleep while you are in the hospital and for the amount of nights you'll be home with a catheter.

✓ **Pain in your throat and difficulty swallowing**. I found sucking on ice chips helped relieve the pain in my throat.

✓ **Gas pain**. You are bloated and need to release gas from both ends. Walking around the unit is the best thing you can do. There is no immediate relief; this takes a lot of time and walking.

Chapter 18

Surgery and My Dreadful Trip Home

The day before surgery is a stressful day. You've been through pre-surgical exams and tests. If you need to travel a long distance to a treatment center, you've had to make arrangements for you and your spouse to stay at a hotel the night before and the night of the surgery, possibly longer. Prior to surgery, you were given a set of written instructions. They included when to stop eating and drinking and when to give yourself an enema.

While I was getting prepped for surgery, another man who was getting prepped for the same surgery admitted to his surgeon he'd eaten solid food within the last twenty-four hours. His surgery was postponed. He had to go home and do everything again at a later date. This lapse in willpower may be hard to admit since doing so will cause a delay in your surgery. However, hiding the fact you ate solid food before surgery could cost you your life (for example, if you eat and then undergo anesthesia, you're at high risk for acid reflux and could choke to death on your own vomit). It's much better to tell your surgeon the truth so you can reschedule your surgery for a time when it will be safe for you to have it.

Before I share my hospital experiences, I want you

to know that I've known many men who were ready, willing, and able to leave the hospital after one night. My experience was different than I expected.

My surgery began at 11:30am. I was brought back to my room around 6:00pm. I expected my pain level would be adequately controlled. It wasn't. My goal the first night was to watch the clock and ask for pain medication as soon as I could get it. It was a very long and pain-filled night.

I noticed two tubes. The first was the catheter; the second was a drainage tube. Neither bothered me the first night. One thing that bothered me was the mechanical stockings on my feet. The sensation was so annoying that I took them off and hid them in the sheets. At the time I had no idea these socks are used to prevent blood clots. Taking them off was a foolish and potentially life-threatening thing to do. Keep them on, no matter how annoying they are. Some hospitals will give men special socks to wear on discharge, and some will not. If you're concerned about this issue or have a history of blood clots, make sure you go home with a pair.

I was fortunate that UCSF allows you to request a private room. Whenever possible, they will honor that request. I appreciated the privacy as well as having family around to visit me. Before I went into the hospital, I was aware that my insurance company had pre-approved a one-night stay in the hospital. My first night following surgery, my pain level was not under control. It was in the seven-to-eight-out-of-ten range. I was in too much pain to sleep. Additionally, I was unpleasantly surprised shortly after breakfast. Within minutes after eating, I went running to the bathroom and deposited my breakfast into the sink. Vomiting after surgery was extremely painful. This event increased my level of pain to its highest point since surgery.

Shortly after vomiting, I was asked if I was ready to go home. I felt pressure to say yes because my insurance company had pre-approved a one-day hospital stay. There was no way I was ready to face a ninety-mile trip home. I needed to stay another night even though I wasn't sure whether my insurance company would cover this additional expense. I'm glad I stayed in the hospital a second night. My insurance company and most insurance companies will cover additional days in the hospital if your surgeon documents the extra days are medically necessary.

On day two, I asked for medication to help with nausea and medication to help me sleep. On night two, I slept well. After taking anti-nausea medication, I kept down lunch, dinner, and then breakfast the following day. My pain level was under control, and I felt ready to leave the hospital.

What I didn't know at the time was how much pain I would experience during the long drive home. Sitting in a car was uncomfortable. Each and every bump on the road caused waves of pain. Within ten minutes on the highway, the pain I felt brought me to tears. I was tempted to ask my son to drive back to UCSF to be readmitted. For the next ninety minutes in the car, I was in excruciating pain. I was sorry I'd left the hospital so soon.

When I got home, I took a sleeping pill and a pain pill. I hoped I could sleep off this episode of pain. Fortunately, I fell asleep. When I woke up, the pain level was manageable. Based on my experiences with my car ride home, here's what I'd do differently:

- ◆ If you have a long drive home, ask for a narcotic pain medication right before discharge.

- ◆ Before you leave the hospital, fill your prescription for your pain medications so it's with you in the car.

- ◆ Have a bottled drink available in case you need to take a pain pill.

- ◆ Buy a donut-shaped pillow for the ride home. You might find it useful the first few days at home as well. I didn't think to buy this pillow, and it hurt so much to sit on our dining room chairs that I ate my meals standing in the dining room. I did this because I wanted to be at the table with my family during dinner. A regular pillow didn't relieve my pain.

It's very important your surgeon writes orders for you prior to surgery. For example, if you are concerned about bladder spasms or nausea, your surgeon can write orders for medication for both issues. If the order is in the chart, you can immediately get medication for the problem. If the order is not in the chart in advance, it's possible you may suffer for hours until your surgeon is contacted.

Things to do:

1. Make a list of things that are important for you to discuss with your surgeon prior to surgery.

2. Make sure you understand the type of pain control you will receive. You do have input in this matter.

3. Ask that orders for anti-nausea medication and bladder spasms be placed in your chart prior to surgery so you can get these medications if you need them.

4. Discuss the possibility of extending your stay in the hospital if it becomes medically necessary.

5. If you purchased black nylon pants with snaps down the side, make sure you wear them for the ride home.

6. Plan for the possibility you won't be comfortable

in bed; have a recliner or an alternate place to sleep prepared for you.

7. If you have any doubts about your ability to sleep with a catheter, make sure you have a prescription for sleep meds for the number of days you'll be living with a catheter.

Chapter 19

Living with a Catheter

Prior to coming home, you should have been given instructions regarding catheter care, as well as other post-surgical instructions and limitations. There is a lot of information to absorb. I suggest you do not receive all this information while you are alone. Have someone with you when you receive your discharge and catheter care instructions.

You made it through surgery, and it's time to come home. If you had a long drive home, I hope the tips you received helped you have a comfortable trip. For the next seven to ten days, you'll be home with a catheter. For a week or two, you will feel very sore. Finding a soft place to sit will be an important task. I was fortunate. We have a reclining chair in our living room and bedroom.

I found it much more comfortable to sleep in a recliner than in a bed. I spent the first two weeks at home sleeping in a recliner. I had a prescription for pills to help me sleep, and I used them each night I slept with a catheter. I was surprised I slept through the night every night with the catheter. It would be many months after the catheter was removed before I'd sleep through the night again. Once the catheter was removed, I needed to use the bathroom every two hours through the night.

You will be provided with two bags—a large bag for nighttime use and a leg bag for going out. This was my sixth time living at home with a catheter, but this would be the longest I'd lived with one. If I'd have known in advance what my life would be like once the catheter was removed, I might have spent more time enjoying the peace rather than counting the days until it would be removed.

For example, if you are unfamiliar with the need for sterilization procedures, you may think this is unimportant, unnecessary, or a waste of time. Nothing could be further from the truth. One mistake can easily lead to a bladder infection, so it's important to follow directions to the letter. I'm going to include a few but not all the important things to know.

Don't ever let your bag get above your bladder. If you do, you run the risk of urine in the bag back flowing into your bladder. This increases the odds of developing a bladder infection, so frequently check your tubes for kinks, and wash the area where the tube enters the penis at least two times a day and after every bowel movement. Call your urologist if you develop any of these symptoms:

- Cloudy urine
- A fever of more than 100.5 degrees or the chills
- Blood present (if there is a lot of blood or a consistent amount of blood, call your doctor)
- If the catheter becomes clogged and you are not draining urine
- If you experience bladder spasms

This list is not all-inclusive, and if you have any questions about catheter care or experience any symptoms that bother you, it's best to call your urologist.

It's extremely important for you to follow all-sterile procedures, including thoroughly washing your hands. I used a hand sanitizer after I washed my hands. It's also important to use the alcohol pads to clean the ends of the bags before changing them. It's time-consuming and a pain in the neck, but it's necessary if you want to avoid a bladder infection.

I did not get along with the small leg bag. It quickly filled with urine. On my first trip out, I filled the bag before I got home. Therefore, it was necessary to go a pubic bathroom to empty my bag. I went into a stall and twisted and turned to find a way to empty the bag into the toilet. It didn't go well. While I emptied the bag, I missed the toilet, and a large amount of the urine spilled directly onto my pants. I was extremely embarrassed. I decided that was the last time I'd wear my leg bag.

I found it advantageous to use the night bag all the time. First, I could be away from home, go to a movie, and not worry about the bag filling up. If the bag got too uncomfortable or heavy to carry because it was filled with urine, I would find a restroom and empty it. Emptying the large bag was easy. There are many men who find life with a catheter fairly easy to cope with. I'm not one of those men. I hated every minute of every day with my catheter. Once I got home, I experienced frequent bladder spasms. This occurs when your bladder attempts to expel the catheter. It was comforting to know my bladder wanted to rid itself of the catheter as much as I did. Bladder spasms can be very painful.

Here were steps I took to use the night bag all the time:

➤ I bought myself baseball pants, the kind that has snaps all along the leg.

➤ I kept one snap open for the tube. You may need to keep the snap open, or it may be possible to snap it closed once the tube is passed through.

➤ I put the large catheter bag in a small plastic shopping bag with a handle, and I carried the bag with me wherever I went. If I was in a restaurant, I'd place the plastic bag under the table. When I walked around the block and spoke to neighbors, no one noticed the catheter. They thought I was carrying a bag with stuff in it.

The good news is your urologist can prescribe medication that will help greatly with bladder spasm pain. Another source of pain came from the tip of my penis. I needed to do two things to reduce this source. First, it was important to make sure the tube was stable and didn't move around while I was walking. The second thing was to apply Lidocaine to the area every few hours.

As soon as you are feeling well enough to leave home, you can take in a movie, go out to eat, or spend some time out of the house to enjoy an activity, even it's a brief walk. I enjoyed walking around the block with my wife and our dog, Teddy.

I'm not one who follows surgical restrictions very well, but there are two you must follow. The first is, even though you may feel capable of driving, you can't as long as you have your catheter.

The second has to do with lifting heavy items. Here again you have the ability, but the consequences could be devastating. In layman's terms, your internal plumbing was disconnected and reconnected. The connections are fragile. Any heavy lifting could damage those connections in such a way that you'd need a catheter for the rest of your life. That awful possibility motivated me to follow my discharge instructions to the letter. Another important way to avoid unnecessary pain is to take the stool softener you will be given. Your rectum will be very sore. Bowel movements and sitting down may hurt for the first few days.

Remember this: once your catheter is removed, it's highly likely you'll be living without urinary control for the next few months. This is one of the most difficult post-surgery issues you'll cope with. Living with a catheter can be unpleasant, but think of this time as the calm before the storm.

Questions to Consider

1. How can you make the best use of your time with a catheter as you recover from surgery?

2. If you can't sleep in a bed, do you have another option?

3. Are there any issues regarding catheter care you are uncertain about? If so, make sure you know who you can call.

4. Is it easy for you to give up driving, or lifting heavy objects, or are you tempted to defy those restrictions?

Chapter 20

Life without a Catheter—Be Careful What You Wish For

The experience with urinary incontinence begins after a much-anticipated event—the day your catheter is removed. I was counting the days. I couldn't wait to rid myself of the ever-present tube in my penis. I never stopped to think about what my life would be like once my catheter was removed. Most men wonder if pulling the catheter out is a painful experience. You feel so vulnerable. Your pants are down, and your penis is showing. There's a tube in your penis that extends into your bladder. You stand in front of the doctor as he or she is about to pull out that tube. This was my experience at my urologist appointment on that day:

Me: How much will this hurt?

Doctor (responds with a joke): It won't hurt *me* a bit.

Before I stopped laughing, the tube was out. The whole experience takes no more than a few seconds. There was very little pain. It's important for you to bring a pad or diaper to this appointment. You may begin leaking urine immediately after your catheter is pulled. I chose to wear a men's adult diaper to the appointment.

I was delighted to be free from my catheter. For a brief

period, it was a happy day. I wanted to celebrate, so I took my wife out for lunch before we headed home. After your catheter is removed, you are also given permission to drive again. I foolishly thought my life was returning to normal once my catheter was pulled. My celebratory mood would last a few brief hours before I experienced an emotional nosedive. I was totally unprepared to deal with the loss of urinary control.

The loss of urinary control is one of the most unpleasant and life-changing side effects of prostate surgery. For men such as myself who have history of benign prostatic hyperplasia (BPH), our prostate was enlarged in such a way as to block the urethra. In order to compensate, the bladder develops muscle tissue to force urine through the blockage. Once your prostate is removed, your bladder continues to respond as if there's a blockage. This problem means it will be more difficult to regain urinary control. As I share my experiences, keep in mind one of the reasons I had so much trouble had to do with my long history with BPH.

I've known a few men who regained their urinary control within hours or days after their catheter was removed. Based on my medical history, I knew in advance I wouldn't be one of those men. Many men I've met through my support groups needed to change three to eight times a day. At first I envied those men. I couldn't understand why they were so upset regarding their circumstances. I would have celebrated to be where they were.

If you are in the majority of men who will lose some degree of urinary control, I can tell you this is an emotionally and physically challenging time. I'm including many unpleasant details of my journey for a specific purpose. I hope you can learn from my mistakes. I made a number of bad decisions that brought needless emotional pain and suffering.

After our celebratory lunch out, my wife and I got home, and I sat on my favorite reclining chair. I leaned back to relax and enjoy living catheter free. I had no idea how much urine I'd leaked in the two hours that had passed since my catheter was pulled. I hadn't the faintest idea how long I could stay in an adult diaper.

Suddenly and unexpectedly, I felt very wet, so I stood up. To my horror and embarrassment, both my jeans and the chair were soaked in urine. I had to wash, change my clothing, and chemically treat the chair so it would not smell. This was my first experience feeling shame, embarrassment and humiliation. These were painful feelings that would become a big part of my life in the days and weeks to come. Since this was my first accident, I quickly got over those feelings. From that time forward, I would place a big pad on the chair so I'd leak on the pad rather than the chair.

Within a few hours, I had the ability to anticipate when I needed to urinate. I was able to quickly start a urine flow. I mistakenly took this as a sign I was regaining urinary control. It wasn't. Other than the one accident on the chair, it was one of the best days I had since my surgery.

Once I was able to drive again, I began taking drives and going places. I began with quick trips. After a few days of successful short trips, I stayed out for longer periods of time. That's when I began to experience public humiliation. I don't know whether my urinary incontinence got worse or that I had no sense of how long I should be in a diaper. Leaking through and wetting my pants in public places soon became the norm. My final humiliation occurred in the mall. My wife and I were enjoying a walk when I suddenly felt my legs getting moist. I happened to look down at my sneakers. They looked like I was caught in the rain. To my horror, I realized urine was dripping down my leg and onto my sneakers. Familiar words I hadn't heard since childhood came to my mind. They came from *Popeye*, a cartoon I watched as a kid. Right before he popped open a can of spinach, he would say (now in a totally different context), "That's all I can stanz, I can't stanz no more."

I went home from the mall and made two decisions. The

first was a healthy decision: I was going to spend whatever time it took to learn how to live in diapers without leaking. The second was not so healthy. I made a vow to stay home until I learned how to manage my diapers in such a way I'd be certain not to have any further public incidents wetting my pants. I made that decision to protect myself from shame and embarrassment. Unfortunately, this vow led to my living as a recluse. I withdrew from friends, my wife, my family, my church family, and my relationship with Jesus. I was in a place where my faith could not impact my thoughts, feelings, attitudes, and behavior. I never stopped believing God would use all of these experiences for my eventual good. I never doubted God's goodness. I was just too discouraged for my faith to make a difference.

I spent the next few weeks doing very little but sitting in my chair feeling sorry for myself. I seriously regretted my decision to have surgery and wondered if I'd ruined my life forever. At that point, if I could have pressed a button that would undo my surgery and get my prostate back, I would have gladly pushed that button—even if I knew the price of pushing the button meant I'd die of prostate cancer. At that point I would have pushed that button without a moment's hesitation.

There was an underlying issue I needed to overcome before I'd stop leaking through my clothes. It had to do with my attitude toward spending money on diapers. My attitude made a bad situation worse, and it seriously affected my emotional well being and my marriage.

I have a history of spending a few hundred dollars every year to purchase the latest and greatest smartphone. There was no way I was going to spend a few hundred dollars per month on diapers and pads. Why would I want to spend the equivalent of a new cell phone each month on a product that ended up in the garbage? I was determined to keep the cost of wearing diapers to a minimum.

This mandate led me to make two decisions that added to my emotional suffering. First, in order to keep costs down, I'd decided to stay in every diaper for three hours. Second, I decided to purchase the cheapest men's diapers I could find. Some of them fit so poorly and were so loose around the legs I now wonder why I wasted valuable time trying to live in poorly made diapers. One time I purchased a cheap package of men's diapers from a national pharmacy. Their brand was so awful and loose fitting that I leaked through, wetting my clothes within thirty minutes. I was so angry that I drove to the pharmacy and said to the clerk, "I know this isn't your fault, but this brand of men's diapers is awful. I couldn't stay dry for thirty minutes. I'd like my money back." She refunded my money. I drove home victorious. It was one of few times I returned poorly fitting diapers. It was highly embarrassing to tell the clerk I was wearing diapers, but the victory of getting my money back made it worth it. Trying to save money by buying cheaply made diapers added extra weeks to the time I'd leak though my diapers.

My second bad decision added more time to this humiliating problem. Most adolescent girls learn the concept of changing their pads based on their blood flow rather than attempt to stay in a pad for a specific number of hours. Unfortunately, I wasn't acting on common sense. I was determined to save money. If I were thinking rationally, I would have made my decision to change my diaper based on how much urine I was leaking rather than how much I was willing to spend on diapers per month.

Even though I was leaking urine through my diaper and onto my clothing a minimum of three times a day, I wouldn't budge. I was sticking to my routine of changing my diaper every three hours no matter how many times a day I leaked through. Rather than reduce the amount of time I'd stay in a diaper, I decided to regulate how much fluid I drank in order to achieve my three-hour goal. Looking back, I regret how stubborn I was about this issue, and how much unnecessary emotional suffering I put myself through in order to save a few dollars.

During this time, my relationship with my body changed. Prior to surgery, I thought of my penis as an organ that gave pleasure to my wife and me. I was surprised when I began thinking of it as my enemy. I was dismayed it was dripping urine all the time. I couldn't walk ten feet from my toilet to the bath without dripping urine on the carpet. It was necessary to place toilet paper over my penis in order to walk a few feet to the bathtub. My constantly dripping penis was ruining my life.

The only time and place I could be free from a diaper was in the shower. Showers became the highlight of my day. Once I came out of the shower, I entered diaper penitentiary. I had a prison nickname for myself. I became "the squirter." Back in elementary school, I read about Dick and Jane. I remember reading, "See Jane run, run, run." Now my story became, "See Rick squirt. Squirt, squirt, squirt." I was regressing and feeling more like a baby than an adult. My entire day was reduced to managing my squirting.

I vividly remember staring at my reflection in the mirror with hatred and contempt as I saw myself wearing a men's diaper. I felt as though I had just journeyed back in time to infancy, except the infant I saw in the mirror had gray sideburns and desperately needed a shave. I said to my reflection, "You are one *big* baby." That's exactly how I felt—like a baby with a man-size bladder.

Nighttime wasn't much better. Because we have a very expensive mattress, we put on a mattress protector. This was a wise decision because there were nights I'd leak through my diaper. By 3:00 a.m. I woke to change my diaper. This involved me turning on the bathroom light, using a wipe, and then changing my diaper and sometimes my pajamas. It usually took an hour or more to get back to sleep. Between 6:00 and 7:00 a.m. I needed another change, and there was no way I could get back to sleep.

I'm certain that sleep disruption affected my mood, energy level, and decision-making abilities in a negative way. Before I was able to successfully gain the skills needed to live in diapers, I had to change my attitude about spending money on them. Unfortunately for my wife, our marriage, and me, it took a few weeks to change my attitude about spending money on diapers. Eventually I came to the place where I began to think of the money I was spending on diapers as a wise investment toward improving the quality of my life. This was a difficult and time-consuming transition to make.

Part of the reason it took so long to do something constructive was because I'd become too depressed to do anything but sit at home and feel sorry for myself. It took me a few weeks before I could motivate myself to experiment with a variety of men's diapers and learn the maximum time I could spend in them without leaking. After experimenting with four different brands, I found one that fit me and worked well. The cost of these adult diapers ran between $.63 and $.75 for each diaper. Once I found the most effective brand, I had to find out how long the diaper could keep me dry. It was obvious three hours was way too long. After many incidents of wetting my pants, I realized it was necessary to change my diaper every hour. That meant going through fifteen to sixteen diapers a day.

The cost of doing this made me crazy. I was spending approximately three hundred forty dollars a month just for diapers. Since I was also using pads, powder, and wipes, the cost moved up to three hundred ninety dollars a month. I'd finally reached a level of desperation where I was willing to spend whatever it took to get some control over urinary incontinence.

I came up with a plan that saved me money and improved the quality of my sleep. I created what I called a "super diaper." I added a men's pad inside my diaper. At 3:00 a.m. I could go to the bathroom, keep the lights out, pull out the pad, throw it away, and stay in the diaper for the rest of the night. This routine made it easier to get back to sleep in the middle of the night. I felt better throughout the day. My mood and decision-making abilities improved. There was one glitch, though. Sometimes the tape from the pad ripped the padding off the front of the diaper. When that happened, I'd end up leaking through the diaper by morning. I learned the hard way if the diaper ripped, I needed to turn on the light, wash up, and change my diaper. After weeks of frustration, isolation, and depression, I was developing the skills to leave the house and come home with dry clothing. It had been a month since I'd laughed or even cracked a smile.

I vividly remember the day my ability to laugh returned. Brenda told me about a Peanuts comic she recently read where Charlie Brown came to the decision to hate one day at a time. The idea of limiting my hatred of my life to one day at a time struck me as both healthy and funny! Until that moment, I didn't hate my life day by day, I was busy projecting my hatred of my life for decades into the future. I decided to model Charlie Brown and learn to hate one day at a time.

This change in thinking had biblical backing. Jesus said in Matthew 6:34, "Therefore do not worry about tomorrow, for tomorrow will worry about its own things. Sufficient for the day is its own trouble."

I felt a significant sense of relief as I kept my hatred of my post-surgical life in the present day rather than extending that hate forward years and decades. Something else happened at the same time. I began to shift my focus and attention away from the things I hated and began to look for and focus my attention on good things that happened each day.

I also noticed that as bad as my worst days were, I survived. I'd finally learned how to manage, live, and cope with severe urinary incontinence. There was no longer a reason to stay home. I could venture out for a few hours with a pad in my diaper. Going out for dinner or to catch a movie was now possible. I had newfound confidence that I could leave the house and come home with dry pants. My wife and I began venturing out into the world, taking in a movie or going out to dinner. We began having fun together. Experiencing fun and pleasure lifted my mood.

I regained access to my faith. I was beginning to learn and grow. The concept of hating one day at a time led me to think about the manna the Jewish people ate in the wilderness. When God provided manna, it was good for a single day. Any attempts to store it for the next day (except for the Sabbath) was met with utter failure. God would supply them with the food they needed for that day and that day only. Then I jumped to the Lord's prayer, where you ask for your daily bread. You don't ask for your allotment of bread for the week, month, quarter, or year.

Then the words of a hymn came to mind: "Morning by morning new mercies I see." My prayers became focused on asking for the grace, mercy, power, and wisdom for each new day. I came to realize God's provisions are for the day. Each and every day it was necessary to ask God for the day's allotment of mercy and grace. I'd also ask for the strength to make it through each new day. I was never let down.

Questions to Consider/ Things to do

1. How are you and your partner preparing for the day your catheter is removed?

2. Discuss how you will feel about losing urinary control. (This will be an ongoing discussion)

Things you can do to prepare:

☐ Have a few different brands of diapers in the house to try (I found Depends to be one of best-fitting brands).

☐ Buy wipes, corn starch, or baby powder

☐ Buy a box of pads to create a "super diaper" (I found Tena pads work great).

☐ Buy a mattress protector

Chapter 21

Learning to Live with Severe Urinary Incontinence

The super diaper (a pad within the diaper) was so effective at night that I wanted to see what would happen if I used it in the daytime. I was willing to leave the house to experiment with my super diaper. I found I could go ninety minutes before it was necessary to find a restroom to rip out the pad. Then I had another ninety minutes before I'd leak in the diaper. I also carried an extra diaper with me wherever I went in case I ripped my diaper when I pulled out the pad. If my diaper ripped, I had to go to a public restroom stall, take off my shoes and pants, and put on a new diaper. Then I had to get dressed, come out of the stall with a urine-filled diaper, and throw it away. This was embarrassing, so I got into the routine of carrying a shoulder bag with pads, diapers, wipes, a change of clothing, and a plastic bag to put my used diaper in so when I left the stall I wasn't seen carrying my diaper to the garbage.

I felt some relief from my depression once I slept more and began leaving the house each day. I did find changing my diaper fifteen times a day took a heavy toll on me physically, emotionally, sexually, and relationally. I still felt as if my life was a nightmare. However, getting out of the house again to go out for a dinner or to a movie was something worth celebrating because I felt like I was slowly returning to the land of the living. If I was out in public with urine-soaked jeans, I felt as though I was carrying a sign that said, "Look at me, I just peed in my pants." When I gave up wearing jeans and switched to dark nylon pants, a spot of urine was not visible to other people. Another advantage of nylon pants was if they got wet from urine, you could go into a restroom to wipe them off. They dried quickly, and soon the wet spot vanished.

In summary, these are these are the lessons I learned the hard way:

> ➢ **Buy the pad or diaper** that works best rather than the cheapest.

> ➢ **Know how long you can stay in a pad or diaper** before needing to change.

> ➢ **Base the need to change on the flow of urine** rather than a function of time or the cost of a diaper. I felt best when I changed my diaper every hour. My suggestion is to start at ninety minutes and work your way up or down depending upon how much urine you are leaking.

> ➢ **Carry a shoulder bag** with a spare set of pants, diapers, pads, wipes, and clothes. Sometimes I kept my bag in my car. At other times, such as at the movies or the mall, I'd carry the bag on my shoulder.

> ➢ **Put away jeans and cotton pants.** Buy dark nylon pants.

> ➢ **Avoid drinking thirty-two-ounce drinks** during your trips away from home.

> ➢ **Most importantly, keep your perspective** (I totally lost mine). For the majority of men, you will regain your urinary control within four months. With all these things in place, I still had some

accidents in public places, but I was well prepared to quickly deal with them. After a few weeks, I had the confidence I needed to leave home for extended periods wearing my diaper.

I was surprised by how long I felt embarrassed about wearing diapers. I felt like a fraud. I was dressed in adult clothing, and from outward appearances, I knew I looked like an adult. That's not how I felt inside. Deep down, I felt like a baby—a baby disguised as an adult. After all, I was still "the squirter." It took me a while to give up my baby nickname and baby identity.

My emotional healing came about after I shared my secret identity with my wife. She reminded me I was man who was diagnosed with prostate cancer. I was a man who chose surgery as the treatment option to treat his cancer. I was a man who was dealing with urinary incontinence, a temporary side effect of surgery. It was through her eyes that my identity transitioned from little baby squirter wearing diapers to a man who needed to wear diapers until I regained urinary control. Reclaiming my adult identity was a victory.

As an adult, I learned how to live and cope with urinary incontinence. Within four months after surgery, I was back in underwear and able to wear jeans and a single pad, which lasted the entire day.

Very few men I've contacted post-surgery needed to change fifteen diapers a day. Yet from my interactions with many men post-surgery, it was obvious they were as distressed as I was, even though they were only changing four to five times a day. I've come to believe the emotional issues involved in dealing with losing urinary control are similar whether you are using four or fifteen diapers a day.

I also discovered the lack of urinary control adversely affected my interest in sex. There was no way I wanted to leak urine on the bed or get naked. Sadly, most men avoid all physical contact with their partners during this time. I fell into this trap as well. I suggest you discuss how urinary incontinence and ED are affecting your interest in sex and all other physical expressions of love and tenderness. In order to avoid dealing with these feelings, it's easy to avoid all forms of physical contact. Sadly, I denied my wife and me of the pleasures associated with kissing, hugging, and holding each other. This decision was a bad one, but I was too depressed to care.

You'll face the following challenges:

♦ Learning to deal with the physical realities of managing pads, diapers, accidents, and incontinence at home and away from home.

♦ Dealing with emotional issues associated with the loss of urinary control.

♦ Discussing with your partner how losing urinary control affects your sexuality and your relationship together.

♦ Balancing the need for support and finding people you can discuss this with against the shame and wanting to keep this a secret from everyone.

Since this is such an unpleasant phase of recovery, it's easy to lose perspective and think, feel and react as though you'll never regain urinary control. It's important to learn to cope with this painfully embarrassing time. It's also important to keep things in perspective. The overwhelming majority of men will experience significant improvement in three months. This phase, while extremely unpleasant, is temporary.

I am not going to go into detail about how to perform Kegels. This is an important exercise you should be taught to perform prior to your surgery. It's believed Kegels will help you regain urinary control. You should not attempt to do them while your catheter is in. There is a significant variation in the number of Kegels patients are told to perform. They range from sixty to a few hundred. I've always believed if a little is good, then more is better, so I started out doing a few hundred Kegels a day. Soon I discovered that too many Kegels caused bladder spasms and fatigue. This meant more leaking rather than less and a significant increase in pain. I settled on six sets of ten per day.

I found an enormous amount of support, comfort, and encouragement through online prostate cancer support groups. It was helpful to speak with men who knew exactly what I was going through.

After four long months, I finally gained control of my bladder. I still needed to wear a pad because I'd still leak urine with sudden movements, while lifting something, or with an unexpected cough or sneeze. After fifteen pads daily, I was grateful for the progress I'd made. If I ended up needing to wear a pad a day for the rest of my life, I'd consider it a blessing.

Approximately seventeen months after surgery, I decided it was time to test whether I could go to work without wearing a pad. I was pleased I'd reached a point where I'd consider trying this. I proudly announced my decision to Brenda. A few minutes before I left the house, I went to the bathroom. I wanted to make sure I had an empty bladder for my five-minute commute to work. I drove to work and parked my car. I got my briefcase, got out of the car, and took two steps.

Suddenly and unexpectedly, I sneezed. I immediately felt myself leak urine. I got to work, went into the bathroom, and confirmed I'd wet my underwear. My reaction to this event was a total surprise. The first thing I did was laugh. I couldn't believe it. I'd just wet my underwear, and I was laughing. The anger, pity, and disgust were all replaced by laughter. It struck me as hilarious that I had performed an experiment to test whether I was ready to live life pad free, and within ten minutes my underwear was wet. Rather than getting discouraged, I was laughing. My ability to laugh about my leaking urine represented a far greater healing than going from fifteen diapers to a pad a day.

At nineteen months post-surgery, I tried this experiment again. This time I went eighteen consecutive days without a single leak! I decided to throw away all my pads. Three weeks later I came down with the flu. With all the coughing and sneezing, I ended up leaking again and needed to wear a pad a day until I recovered. It was no big deal to go back to wearing a pad. The emotional trauma associated with urinary incontinence was gone forever.

Questions to Consider

1. How are you managing your accidents?

2. Are there things you can learn to make this time less difficult?

3. How is urinary incontinence affecting your marriage?

4. How has urinary incontinence affected your sex life?

5. How is losing urinary control affecting your self-esteem, and your mood?

6. Have you learned what you need to know about living in diapers, or are you wetting your pants multiple times per day?

7. Do you have the support you need to get you through this very unpleasant time in your life? If not, I suggest you visit our post-surgery forum at **whereisyourprostate.com**.

Chapter 22

Your Pathology Report

A few days after surgery, you will receive your pathology report. Think of your prostate as a walnut wrapped in several layers of plastic wrap. The walnut is close to the average size of a prostate. The plastic wrap covering the walnut is like the multi-layered membrane that covers your prostate. Once your prostate is removed, it goes to a pathologist.

After testing, you will receive valuable information about your cancer. They will tell you if your cancer is contained within the prostate, or in and outside your prostate but contained in the prostate membrane (the plastic wrap). This is called specimen-confined.

Cancer cells may be out of the membrane. This is called positive surgical margins.

Lastly and more seriously is when cancer cells are found in other places, such as your seminal vesicles or a lymph node.

I'll never forget the way I was given the news. I received a phone call from UCSF. The doctor began by saying the pathology report he was about to share was a dream report that every prostate cancer patient wants to receive. I was already joyful before he shared the specifics. He went on to tell me my cancer was downgraded from 3+4 to 3+3.

I was also told my cancer was totally confined within my prostate. With early detection, a higher percentage of men are receiving the similar news. It is fantastic news to learn your cancer was confined within the prostate.

From the other direction, I've also met a surprising number of men who received the news their cancer had spread. Receiving this news is more devastating than the original diagnosis. Those of us who chose surgery were hoping and perhaps expecting surgery to be the final solution and cure for our prostate cancer. It's hard to go through surgery and then receive the bad news cancer cells were found in other locations. In all likelihood, this means there's a need for additional treatment. From an emotional standpoint, there are a number of things going on. First, many men are still struggling with urinary incontinence and impotence. Then you receive the news that your hopes for a surgical resolution for prostate cancer have been dashed on the rocks.

If you receive this news after surgery, you might feel any of the following emotions:

❖ Feeling overwhelmed with life. First you heard about the diagnosis of cancer, and then you had the trial of choosing a treatment option. Now you're coping with the aftermath of surgery, only to find out cancer cells are in other places in your body.

❖ There is the profound sense of disappointment that surgery didn't remove all the cancer cells.

❖ There is a heightened sense of fear of the cancer spreading and leading to an early death.

❖ There is an increase in anxiety about what to do next, how effective the next form of treatment will be, and the additional side effects of the next treatment options.

❖ There may be a sense of futility about coping

with the aftermath of surgery knowing it didn't have the expected results.

❖ A pervasive sense of pessimism about the future may occur, as it appears that things have gone from bad to worse.

❖ You may be angry about the circumstances you are facing.

Now is the time you'll need the support of your entire team, yet the stress of this illness may have taken a toll on your relationship. If your marriage was stressed before the diagnosis of cancer or your history of problem solving is poor, you may experience an increase in fighting and emotional and physical distance from one another. If you are able, put hurts and resentments on the shelf right now. Deal with them at a later time. Now is the time to be kind, thoughtful, considerate, and supportive of one another.

Sit down together and begin sharing what this journey of dealing with prostate cancer has been like for each of you. Talk about your fears, frustrations, and disappointments. Make time to share your love for one another. Spend a lot of time doing that.

If you find yourself angry about choosing surgery and dealing with all the changes that came with it, know this: your surgery gave you important information you would not have known otherwise. Assuming your cancer has spread, you have the opportunity to treat it in ways that can extend your life expectancy. Remember this: if you did not have the surgery, you would never have known how serious your prostate cancer was. You had the skills and ability to choose surgery as your treatment option. As a result of this wise choice, you've learned there's more to do. You've made it this far. This means you have the ability to use these next few weeks to read, do research, and speak with doctors and other men who've faced this dilemma. Eventually you will decide what you will do next to continue fighting the battle against cancer.

Rely on each other and your team during this highly stressful time in your life. Don't neglect each other. Take time to enjoy your life. Find things to do as a couple. Pray together often. Make sure you make room in your life for laughter and love. Last, prepare yourself for battle. Your fight against this disease is not over. A new battle has begun. For me, the battle with cancer was over.

Here are some questions/ ideas to consider:

1. Begin by talking about some things you love and/ or appreciate about each other.

2. Take the time to talk to your spouse about how you both feel about the news you received after surgery.

3. What are your biggest fears?

4. What are you frustrated about?

5. Who will you need to consult in order to decide what to do next?

6. How can you get the support you need to get through this difficult phase?

Chapter 23

Living with Bladder Spasms

Some men will experience bladder spasms after surgery. Mine began within the first forty-eight hours after surgery. During my spasms, I noticed urine leaking around the catheter tube. Nursing staff explained this often occurs during spasms.

It's hard to describe what spasms feel like since people experience different sensations, sometimes in different places. Some describe spasms as a cramping feeling. I experienced a burning sensation and painful contraction at the tip of my penis. You may feel pressure in your pelvic region or in your rectum. Bladder spasms are unpleasant and may be quite painful.

Years ago I was diagnosed with interstitial cystitis. As a result, I had a history with bladder spasms and pelvic floor spasms prior to my prostate surgery. This meant I was at a higher risk than most to suffer through this. Removing the catheter did not stop my spasms. They continued on for many months. Most men's spasms will end within the first month. Many men won't experience them at all.

If you do experience bladder spasms, there are a few triggers you can control. One is changing your diet. You will need to avoid the following because they can irritate the lining of your bladder:

- Citrus foods and drinks, such as oranges or orange juice
- Spicy foods
- Alcohol
- Tomatoes
- Chocolate
- Caffeinated beverages, including coffee, tea, and colas

Another thing to do is avoid a full bladder. Try to urinate every hour and increase your fluid intake. From my personal experience, one recommendation to help with spasms actually triggered them. While I was doing a set of ten Kegels, I'd often start to spasm. When I stopped the Kegels, the spasms stopped, so I'd wait a few hours before I'd do another set.

If you've taken these steps listed above and are still experiencing spasms, there is no reason to tough this out. If you are experiencing bladder spasms, call your urologist, explain the steps you've taken, and ask for medication. I've read many threads on prostate cancer forums where men have called their urologists about painful spasms but were not offered medication. If your urologist does not want to prescribe medication to treat your spasms, find out why. If you are not satisfied with the explanation, I'd suggest you see another urologist for a second opinion.

I experienced my most embarrassing incident with a bladder spasm after my catheter was removed. I was in a public restroom standing in front of the urinal. As I began my flow, I was hit with a painful bladder spasm. I was knocked off my feet. As I began to fall, I noticed I wasn't able to stop my flow. I fell to the floor, urinating as I fell. I made quite a mess. I was grateful I was alone in the bathroom. For the next few months, any time I had to urinate in public, I used a stall and sat down. There was no way I was willing to give a repeat performance of that event in a restroom filled with other men.

I found the medication I was prescribed to be highly effective in stopping my spasms. The only downside to taking medication was the experience of having a dry mouth, but I preferred a dry mouth to experiencing bladder spasms.

I have an embarrassing confession to make: I didn't follow my own advice. After I finished my prescription for bladder spasms, the spasms continued, and I decided I'd tough it out rather than call for a refill. I suffered from daily spasms until I went to UCSF eleven months post-surgery to discuss why my penile injections had stopped working. While I was there, I mentioned this problem and received medication. My spasms went away within twenty-four hours. Suffering needlessly for ten months was a foolish choice, especially when I knew better. Sometimes men do stupid things.

Chapter 24

What's Sleep Got to Do with It?

There are a number of places during this journey where you could experience serious sleep disruption. Here are some of the high-risk areas for losing sleep for a consecutive number of days.

❖ After receiving the news of a lump or a rise in PSA

❖ After you receive the news you have prostate cancer

❖ After you discover how much you need to learn in order make a treatment decision

❖ Waiting four to six weeks for surgery

❖ Dealing with post-surgical pain at home

❖ Sleeping with a catheter after surgery

❖ Living in diapers and feeling wet at night

❖ Having to get up to urinate multiple times during the night

❖ Dealing with long-term erectile dysfunction

Based on my previous experiences with a catheter, I thought my worst experience would be the nights I slept in a reclining chair. With the aid of prescription medication, I slept better in the recliner with a catheter than I did the next six months in bed without one. Once the catheter was removed, I experienced significant sleep disruption due to living in diapers and coping with severe urinary incontinence. The first three months after my catheter was pulled, I went to bed every night at 11:00 p.m. I got up to urinate at 1:00 a.m., 3:00 a.m., 5:00 a.m., and finally at 7:00 a.m., when I'd get out of bed and start the day. Each time I'd wake up, it took me thirty minutes to an hour to fall back asleep.

Looking back, I believe sleep deprivation played a significant role in affecting my mood, my decision-making abilities, and my tolerance for frustration. There are a number of potential consequences of persistent sleep disruption. I've experienced all of these symptoms:

1. Poor cognitive functioning (you won't think as well, problem solve, or react to situations appropriately)

2. Easily irritated (you will get ticked off at minor events)

3. Lack of energy

4. Binge eating and weight gain

5. Depression

6. Falling asleep at inappropriate times

7. Difficulty remembering things

8. Prone to illness

9. An exaggerated sense of pain

Without proper sleep, a difficult journey becomes even more difficult. If at any point in this journey you have consecutive nights you are unable to sleep, I have a few suggestions. First, take time early in the day to process things that are upsetting to you. Avoid the following a few hours before you go to bed:

➤ Caffeinated drinks

➤ Your computer and TV

➤ Stop drinking all liquids

➤ Smoking

➤ Make sure you have a comfortable pillow and mattress.

➤ Spend time praying before falling asleep.

➤ Pick a regular time each night to fall asleep.

If you experience chronic difficulty with constant fatigue, falling asleep, staying asleep, or snoring, consult your physician. You may have sleep apnea, or you might need medication for a period of time in order to get a good night's sleep. Good sleep is vital to your recovery after surgery. Don't ignore the importance of sleeping well. Getting a good night's sleep is essential to both your physical and psychological health. The lack of sleep will affect your capacity to cope with the emotional upheavals of your post-surgical life.

Questions/Thoughts to Consider

1. Is it taking you longer to fall asleep while you are living in diapers? If so, should you consider the possibility of prescription sleep aides until you no longer need diapers?

2. How many times during the night are you waking up? Would a "super diaper" (a diaper with a pad) increase the amount of time you could sleep?

3. Is the lack of sleep affecting you in any way? (In

order to get accurate information you need to ask your family this question)

4. What steps can you take that will improve the amount of hours you sleep in a day? (For example, would taking an afternoon nap help?)

Chapter 25

Let's Not Get Physical—
Why Men Give Up Sex

I found it difficult to enjoy sex after surgery. My erectile abilities were gone. Orgasms without erections were so diminished in intensity that at times I wasn't even sure I had one. My desire for sex completely disappeared, and I wondered why. More than that, I wanted to understand when and why this had happened. One year after surgery, I had some answers.

Many men report a noticeable reduction in their libido sometime following surgery. A noticeable drop in my interest in sex began shortly after my urologist felt a lump in my prostate. After I received my biopsy results, my sex drive plummeted to the lowest level of my life. A year after surgery my interest in sex remained greatly diminished. There are so many reasons this could happen. I'll give a few from my life. Emotional upheaval can reduce the desire for sex. I experienced significant levels of fear and anxiety prior to the diagnosis of cancer and even higher levels once the diagnosis was confirmed.

After surgery, a combination of post-surgical issues came together in a perfect storm taking away my desire for sex. I considered experience of ejaculation to be extremely pleasurable. The loss of ejaculation combined with the diminished intensity of my orgasm resulted in my feeling disappointed rather than satisfied. I lost the capacity to enjoy my orgasms. Rather than feeling satisfied after my orgasms, I felt terribly sad. Sex became something I wanted to avoid, because all the familiar physical pleasures associated with sex was absent from the experience. I had no idea if or when I'd ever enjoy my sexuality ever again.

If all that wasn't enough to destroy my sex drive, there is another major issue to face after surgery called erectile dysfunction. I lost my ability to achieve an erection. You don't realize the meaning of erections until you lose that ability.

> Erections were a reminder from my body that a sexual release would be greatly enjoyed.

> Erections served as a signal that I was aroused.

> Erections served as a reminder to meet my wife's emotional needs.

> Erections affirmed my manhood.

> Erections enabled me to experience physical intimacy and satisfy my wife sexually as well as myself.

After I lost my ability to achieve an erection, I felt like a eunuch. Losing the ability to achieve an erection is a physical symptom. ED also affected me emotionally, psychologically, and relationally. How you feel about yourself, your wife, and your marriage changes once you lose your erectile abilities. I think my reaction to erectile dysfunction was fairly typical. For a host of reasons I wanted to avoid sex at all costs. Sadly, once I took this position, I also gave up expressing all forms of affection, including hugging, holding hands, and kissing. All of it stopped.

It took no effort to maintain this decision because my desire for sex, which prior to surgery was strong, was now nonexistent. It was somewhere around four weeks post-surgery when I had my first orgasm with a flaccid penis.

As this was happening, I suddenly began squirting fluid. I was told ejaculations would not be possible, yet there I was ejaculating! Somehow, some way, I thought I had gotten a lucky break. I was totally filled with joy. It only took a few seconds before my joy turned into disgust when I realized I was urinating, not ejaculating. I urinated on my bed sheets and on my wife. The shame and humiliation I felt was beyond words.

In his book *Saving Your Sex Life: A Guide for Men with Prostate Cancer*, Dr. John Mulhall reported approximately 90 percent of men who have surgery will have this experience at least once. I'm in the 20 percent of the men who will experience this as an ongoing problem. The medical term for this condition is "climacturia," which is the involuntary release of urine at the time of orgasm during sexual activity. No one ever mentioned the possibility I'd experience this issue following surgery. It's highly likely no one will mention it to you either. It's an awful, romance-killing issue that continues to plague me nineteen months after surgery. It's a very unpleasant and highly embarrassing issue to discuss with anyone. Who wants to tell their doctor, " I am urinating, before, and during my orgasms."

I've come to believe there is a "don't ask, don't tell" conspiracy of silence when it comes to this problem. Your doctor may not ask, and you'll be too embarrassed to tell. The first few months following surgery I'd leak urine during foreplay. I'd leak when I experienced throbbing during bursts of excitement, and I'd urinate during my orgasm. It was bad enough I couldn't attain an erection. Leaking urine fueled my sense of shame and humiliation. If you experience this problem, I encourage you to discuss this with your doctor and your partner. Eventually, I realized going to the bathroom right before my orgasm, while not romantic, significantly reduced the volume of urine I'd squirt. I also discovered lying on my back during my orgasm significantly reduced the amount of urine I'd leak. Nineteen months post-surgery I still leak a small amount of urine. The majority of men will grow out of this symptom in a few months.

I am blessed to have a wife who was amazingly supportive rather than repulsed by this problem. We have a mattress pad to protect our mattress, and I keep a towel on our bed to deal with my urine leaks. Sadly, in the beginning and for a few months, I could not accept my wife's understanding or support. My sense of shame ran too deep. I wanted to avoid all attempts at intimacy until this symptom improved. I discovered it was more than shame that fueled my withdrawal from sexual intimacy. There was also a shift in my relationship to my body. Prior to surgery, my penis and I were on very friendly terms. I thought of this organ as a source of tremendous pleasure. Shortly after my catheter was pulled, my perpetually leaking penis became the enemy that was ruining my life. As my enemy, I sentenced my penis to an indefinite long-term stretch of solitary confinement. That place of isolation happened to be in my adult diaper.

As judge and jury, I determined my penis would never see the light of day, nor would it be touched again until it stopped the continual dripping of urine. Looking back, I didn't just sentence my penis to solitary confinement, I sentenced my wife and myself. What I didn't know at the time was waiting until I achieved urinary control was not going to solve this issue. I wrongly assumed that once I regained bladder control, I'd have the same control during sex. Sadly, this wasn't the case.

There was another emotion I was trying to avoid. I still had a significant amount of sadness and grief over the things I had lost with regard to my sexuality. Here's my list of things that cause me grief:

➢ The loss of ejaculation

➢ The lessening of intensity of my orgasms

➢ The fact that in every phase of excitement, I leak urine

➢ My penis remains flaccid no matter how excited I am

➢ After each orgasm, rather than feeling pleasure or satisfied, I'd feel profoundly sad as I compared my pre-surgery sex life with my post-surgery sex life.

➢ I wondered if my sex life was ruined forever.

➢ I was angry I had cancer. I was angry I wasn't one of the men who regained erectile abilities. I was angry about the changes prostate surgery brought to my sex life.

➢ I worried whether I'd suffer permanent damage to my erectile tissue and lose the ability to have erections ever again. I was also worried about the loss of my sex drive. I worried that my interest in sex would never return.

➢ Fear loomed large. I was fearful I'd never enjoy sex again. I was afraid my sense of manhood was damaged beyond repair.

➢ Disappointment was ever present. I was disappointed with the quality and intensity of my orgasms. From start to finish, the whole sexual experience was disappointing.

It's impossible to enjoy your sexuality when so many negative emotions intrude on the experience. You or your partner may have other emotions you want to add to my list. I suggest both of you write your list of unpleasant feelings that have invaded your sexual relationship and discuss each one, without getting angry or defensive. When (notice I said when, not if) anger or defensiveness becomes evident, rather than giving in to those feelings, observe them and ask yourself what it is about this issue that makes it so difficult to talk about. Deal with that resistance before you go back to dealing with the issue that brought out the anger or defensiveness.

Any one of the unpleasant thoughts or emotions

listed above could have a negative impact on your sexual relationship in a major way. I was feeling all of the above. It's enough to make one or both of you throw up your hands and give up on the possibility of enjoying sex together ever again. If you don't make that decision outright, it may come by default. If you choose to avoid dealing with your multiple losses and unpleasant feelings, it's possible you'll do what I did, which was avoid sex in every form. This means every form of affection is given up and avoided. Looking back, I deeply regret my decision to act in this way. I added to my own personal suffering. Even worse, I added to Brenda's suffering. You can attempt to push those unpleasant feelings away or bury them underground, but they will not go away. The stress, fighting, emotional distance, and unhappiness in your marriage are symptoms of avoiding the losses you face with your sexuality.

Some important lessons I learned during this phase:

♦ In order to come to a place where I could enjoy my new sexuality, I had to grieve and say good-bye to my old sexuality. This process takes time. I had to be willing to face my sadness with each and every orgasm and mourn the loss of my pre-surgery sexuality.

♦ I couldn't sit on the sidelines and wait two years for my nerve bundles to heal and for erections to return in order to enjoy my sexuality. I could be proactive. The next chapter on penile rehabilitation will talk about the steps that can be taken.

♦ I had to find a new definition of manhood that wasn't dependent on my erectile abilities and performance in the bedroom.

♦ I had to learn how to appreciate other forms of physical affection without getting frustrated they didn't excite me the same way they used to. This lesson was difficult to learn.

♦ I had to learn ways to cope with uncontrolled

urination during each phase of sex. I learned to trust God and involve Him in this struggle. I knew there were important lessons to learn about my sexuality and my manhood that would only come from God.

♦ I learned I could not cope with this alone, and I needed to speak to men online who were coping with similar experiences.

♦ I learned how important it is to discuss my feelings and my fears with my wife rather than deal with them alone.

♦ I learned real men don't lose their masculinity based on the state of their penis. Real men face their struggles and trials head on.

♦ Manhood involves the willingness to get help when you need it.

♦ Long-term trials have the potential to develop an important character trait called perseverance.

♦ Manhood involves learning how to act in loving ways even when it's tough to do so. If a man doesn't know how to do this, he is willing to learn how. In other words, men willing to grow must have a teachable spirit.

As this learning was occurring, I issued my penis a judicial pardon. The sentence of solitary confinement was commuted. The judicial pardon was issued even though my penis still leaked urine. It was now free to leave diaper penitentiary. I thought I was ready to find ways to explore a satisfying sex life with the new realities and losses that were present as a result of prostate surgery.

This road had more bumps than I could have imagined. Prior to surgery, you might wonder why on earth the search for pleasure would be difficult. Sex with a flaccid penis is different than sex with an erect penis. Erections have decades of associations with sexual interest, tension, and excitement. A flaccid penis has no such associations. It is strange to build up excitement when your penis remains flaccid. A flaccid penis is associated with the lack of interest and excitement. I had to make brand-new connections in my mind in order to enjoy, build, and experience sexual tension without an erection.

If that wasn't difficult enough, the entire sequence of building tension and increasing excitement leading to an explosion of ejaculate was changed in ways that weren't recognizable. In fact, for me and for many men, the quality and intensity of the orgasmic experience was greatly diminished. I learned how to accept and listen to all the unwelcome emotions and thoughts that followed every orgasmic experience. Everything familiar about my sexuality was gone. The loss of urinary control and erectile abilities are two significant losses that assault your identity as a man. My feelings of regret and buyer's remorse for choosing surgery were at their highest levels at this time.

Coping with these changes is difficult and challenging in a healthy marriage. Facing these issues in a stressed marriage can result in increased fighting, a sharp drop in marital satisfaction, and thoughts of ending your relationship. This is why I suggested you get a marital tune-up or seek professional help before facing these painful struggles. If you did not follow that advice, it may be necessary for you to do this now during this extremely stressful phase of recovery. It also means you will need to discuss the very difficult topic of what has happened to your sexual relationship since surgery.

The idea of discussing sexual issues with a stranger is difficult. For many couples, it's so humiliating that it's easier for men to choose to ignore or neglect their sexuality and their wives' sexuality than to seek professional help. For some couples, divorce is a preferable option to suffering through the embarrassment and humiliation of seeking help and discussing highly intimate details of their lives. I believe this task would be easier for men if surgeons stepped up to the plate and inquired about the problem men have with their sexuality after surgery. Unfortunately, most surgeons do not receive much training on how to discuss these issues, so men continue to suffer in silence and alone. Their partners suffer as well.

The decision to avoid sex brings pain, hurt, frustration, and a loss of goodwill in the best of marriages. In stressed marriages, these problems could rapidly lead to an affair or a divorce. I believe it's a huge mistake to cope with these issues alone or end a marriage rather than seek help. Sex after a prostatectomy is not the same as sex before surgery. There are losses to be grieved. Couples do better when they can help each other through a grieving process. It's important for men to remember their partners are also grieving. You're not the only one facing loss. This is a time to draw closer to each other and to God.

The loss of erectile abilities does not give you an excuse to withdraw from your wife emotionally or sexually. Sadly, that is exactly what I did. Suffering from severe depression can make it difficult, if not impossible to act in loving ways. If you find you are sad or hating your life for the majority of your waking hours, it is time to get some help from either a support group and/or a professional. Your surgeon, treatment center, or pastor may have sources of support for you and your partner. Given all you are dealing with, there is no shame in admitting you can't cope with this alone.

My wife was an amazing source of support, and so was my faith, but neither of these two pillars of support prevented me from sinking into a deep, dark depression. My wife reminded me that her perspective regarding sex was very different from mine. For most women, sex includes all types of affection—holding hands, giving back rubs, hugging, kissing, cuddling, etc. Last I checked, none of these activities felt any different or less pleasurable after surgery. While erections were a big part of intimacy prior to surgery, now a couple must work to find other ways to satisfy one another. This is where one has to get creative and perhaps step out of your prior sexual history or comfort zone. It is possible for a man to satisfy his partner without an erection? Ask your partner how she'd like you to continue to satisfy her sexually.

You still have powerful parts of your body that can work to provide sexual satisfaction—arms, hands, fingers, mouth, and tongue. Some couples find oral sex disgusting while others find it extremely enjoyable. Sex toys, such as vibrators or many other options, can also provide enjoyment for both partners. If you are too shy to buy these items in a store, they can be purchased privately online. This is a time to get creative and imaginative. While the experience wasn't as intense, I learned over the course of time to enjoy orgasms without erections. Each couple will be challenged to use their imagination and creativity to find ways for a man to obtain and enjoy sexual satisfaction after surgery.

The question for each couple becomes, how will you wait for the next eighteen to twenty-four months for your nerve bundles to heal? Some men decide if they can't have a whole loaf and enjoy sex the way they did prior to surgery, they'd rather withdraw and forget about it. I vacillated back and forth. Sometimes I was able to enjoy our sexual relationship. Other times I avoided sex and all forms of physical intimacy.

I am still struggling with the idea that a half a loaf is infinitely better than no loaf. It isn't easy or natural for me to come to that conclusion. Sometimes I'm grateful for how far I've come. At other times I get seriously discouraged and/or depressed about the permanent losses surgery has brought to my sexuality. Without purposeful effort, erectile dysfunction can ruin or destroy your relationship. It's important for couples to find ways to make their physical time together emotionally and physically pleasurable. This became less difficult when I experienced a return of the intensity of my orgasms approximately ten months following surgery.

I have no idea whether I'll experience spontaneous

erections ever again, though I hope I will. At sixteen months it takes ED medication and direct penile stimulation to experience an erection. I'm able to experience some degree of hardness and a useable erection for a brief period. I enjoy my orgasms without the intrusion of grief, sadness, and loss. I do not avoid physical touch, such as kissing, holding hands, or lying in each other's arms. Unfortunately, my desire and interest in sex remains greatly diminished. I have no idea whether this is a permanent change. If it is, I can live with it.

My nurse practitioner at UCSF told me the nerve bundles continue healing through the third year post-surgery. I have to wait another year before I'll know how surgery permanently impacted my erectile abilities. In the meantime, I'm grateful to live in an era were ED medication is available. It is still frustrating that reliable and useable erections are still a hit or miss experience. For now, we make the best of what we have. I suspect that's a good lesson to learn, because it's not only surgery that brings about loss; the process of aging does that on its own.

Sexual healing is not a return to my pre-surgery levels of interest, excitement, or enjoyment. It's an acceptance to give and receive what's available to enjoy. It's been a rough road to make peace with the changes in my sexuality following surgery. It may be a rough road for you as well.

Questions/Thoughts to Consider

1. How easy is it for you to talk about your sexual relationship?

2. How satisfying was your sexual relationship prior to surgery? (If the answer is not very, things may get progressively worse after surgery.)

3. Share with your partner the things you currently enjoy about your sexual relationship.

4. How important is it for you to maintain your current level of sexual activity?

5. How will a reduction in sexual activity affect you?

6. How flexible are you with regard to finding other ways to obtain mutual sexual satisfaction?

7. Develop plans to enjoy your physical life together during the phase in which erectile dysfunction will be part of your life.

8. Talk about the ways in which surgery may alter your sex lives permanently.

Chapter 26

Looking for Love in All the Wrong Places

It's my prayer that you will read this chapter and stay clear of these places. Erectile dysfunction brought about an overwhelming sense of desperation. This can lead to a decision to step outside the boundaries of marriage to see whether novel experiences will kick-start your interest in sex or help you experience a more intense form of arousal.

The temptation to use pornography, have an affair, or seek out a prostitute may cross your mind. For some men, fighting this temptation will be extremely difficult to overcome, especially if they are the ones highly interested in maintaining a sex life, but their partners are turned off by leaking urine or their inability to have an erection. Working through these issues is difficult, especially for couples who are highly embarrassed, or have no previous history of talking about sexual issues with each other.

Making one of these choices is a danger sign that you are looking for love in all the wrong places:

❖ Using illegal drugs to alter your mood.

❖ Drinking alcohol in order to forget or feel better.

❖ Participating in compulsive sexual activity, like masturbating frequently.

❖ Watching X-rated movies or viewing pictures of people performing sexual acts or posing in provocative ways.

❖ Using an activity to escape an unpleasant reality. This can include spending too many hours watching TV, playing games on the Internet, shopping, or a host of other activities designed to help us escape or distract us from facing our circumstances.

❖ Giving up on the idea of receiving comfort and deciding to isolate from everyone. (Often this is the first step toward pornography addiction).

I found I could easily rationalize viewing pornography. My rationalization went something like this: by using pornography, I'm not attempting to cheat on my wife. My goal is to help me obtain an erection so my wife and I can enjoy a sexual experience together. As rationalizations go, I thought mine was a good one. Thankfully, I realized that using porn would be dangerous. I knew that if I began to use images of other women in order to become excited or attain an orgasm, I'd be training myself to need that type of imagery. I did not want to become dependent on the use of pornography. Once you bring it into your sex life, it's difficult to give up.

It became clear to me how important it was for my wife to be the only woman involved with the rebirth of my sexuality. I did not want to put myself in the position of needing to see other women in order to get excited. I confessed to my wife the struggle I had with the temptation to use pornography and affirmed my commitment to her. I missed the days when touching her, seeing her, and kissing her would easily bring about an erection. I had to remember it wasn't just the surgery that brought changes in my responsiveness. I wasn't in my twenties anymore; I was rapidly approaching sixty. Prior to surgery, the process of aging brought on some unwelcome changes in my libido and decreased my responsiveness. Unfortunately, surgery took these changes to another level.

Between my inability to obtain an erection and the issue of leaking urine, I was determined to avoid all physical contact with Brenda. I turned to two familiar places for escape and distraction. The first was the TV. I wanted to watch as much TV as possible so I wouldn't have to think about things. The second source of distraction was my trusty laptop. I could easily spend a few hours a day online. Between the TV and the computer, I spent the majority of my waking hours at home in front of one screen or the other. While these distractions had some value, my emotional pain still remained.

I knew I needed to find additional sources of emotional comfort. Sadly, rather than turning to my wife or my faith, I turned to food. I began to eat lots of junk food. Prior to my surgery, I'd lost twenty-three pounds. My waist went down to size thirty-six. My goal was to reach size thirty-four. For the first time in many years, I was feeling good about my body. I wanted to lose another twenty pounds.

During the four months I struggled with severe urinary incontinence, I gained back all twenty-three pounds. Now I had another reason to avoid sex—I hated the way I looked and felt at two hundred twenty pounds. I also had another reason to keep eating: food gave me temporary comfort and relief from self-loathing. It was a vicious cycle. My waist size went from size thirty-six to back to size thirty-eight. As I continued to gain weight, wearing size thirty-eight pants became uncomfortable, but that's what I wanted. I didn't feel I deserved to be comfortable in clothing. I wanted my clothing to give me physically painful reminders that I was overweight. When I looked in the mirror, I was disgusted. I looked similar to how my wife looked when she was nine months pregnant. The last thing I needed in life was another reason to hate myself. Unfortunately for me, that's exactly what happened.

Reasons to hate myself—let me count the ways:

❖ I wasn't responding sexually as a man.

❖ I couldn't stop leaking urine.

❖ I couldn't control my impulse to overeat.

❖ Physically, I looked awful. I hated the way I looked.

There was no hope of bringing my eating under control until I was willing to face the issues I was stuffing down by eating. Here's what didn't work:

❖ Trying to develop more willpower

❖ Skipping meals

❖ Depriving myself of my favorite foods.

❖ Hating myself into a healthy body.

How we speak to ourselves may change after surgery. We can become a cruel judge and jury over ourselves. If this happens to you, you'll notice how harshly you think about your body, your sense of manhood, your role as a husband and lover, or your sexuality.

We say harsh things to ourselves, like:

❖ I'm no longer a man.

❖ I have no value.

❖ My wife would be better off without me.

❖ I'm useless in the bedroom.

If we try to avoid dealing with the emotional pain or harsh judgments we've made about ourselves, we will find a legal or illegal drug, an addiction, or some activity to numb our pain.

Here are some examples of how grace and truth spoke to the issues that bothered me. About my weight, I told myself, "Yes, you blew it and gained a lot of weight. You've got a great exercise routine going; keep that up. No more starving yourself or skipping meals. I don't have to feel hunger pangs in order to lose weight. I can eat things I enjoy, but I'll need to pay attention to the portion size of those things if I'm going to lose weight. I'll need to deal with difficult and painful emotions rather than stuffing them down with food. I need to be kind and loving to myself rather than harsh and critical."

About my sexuality, I had to challenge the notion I couldn't be a real man with a flaccid penis. I also had to challenge my all-or-nothing way of thinking. My unhealthy self-talk went like this: "If I can't have an erection, I'll avoid all forms of affection." My healthy self-talk went like this: "Sure, things aren't the way you'd like them to be, but all is not lost. There's a lot I'm able to enjoy. Touching, kissing, holding hands, and stroking each other are all very pleasant. I deserve to enjoy those things."

My wife and I are open and flexible regarding our sex lives. We found enjoyable ways to satisfy one another. After many months, it became clear that no option available was going to give me a reliable erection. It took a while to reach the point where I was determined not to put my sexuality on hold or on the shelf while I waited for my nerve bundles to heal. My wife and I had a romantic getaway eleven months after surgery. ED medication totally failed, yet we had a wonderful time. Without the grace, love, and truth that came from my faith, I would have turned to pornography and fantasy rather than to my loving and exciting wife. Needless to say, it's important for every man and every couple to look and find love in all the right places. Every man can make that commitment. That's what real men do.

> ➤ They stay faithful to their wives and wedding vows.

> ➤ They consider their partners' needs as seriously as their own.

> ➤ They know that sexuality involves more than erections and orgasms.

> ➤ They demonstrate affection to their partner verbally and physically.

> ➤ Their self-worth and value comes from their character rather than their sexual performance.

> They base their self-esteem on God's view of them rather than their sexual abilities.

<u>Questions/Thoughts to Consider</u>

1. Take time and write down some of the harsh things you've thought about yourself since surgery.

2. What has happened to your sense of manhood since you've lost your erectile abilities?

3. Are you numbing your pain with alcohol, drugs, pornography, food, or anything else?

4. Are you willing to give up all of the above in order to deal with the emotional pain you are feeling?

5. If you are unable to stop any activity, which is numbing your pain, are you willing to get professional help? If not, why not? Ask your partner the price your relationship will suffer if you refuse to get help.

6. How can you help each other face the painful emotions you both feel?

7. How can your faith help you re-define your concept of manhood, so it isn't dependent upon your sexual prowess?

Chapter 27

Battling Sadness, Loss, Grief, and Depression

If you are one of those fortunate men who regain urinary control and erectile function shortly after your catheter is removed, you are less likely to suffer from depression. If you aren't depressed post-surgery, skip down to the section that deals with sadness and loss. If you are unhappy with your life post-surgery or thinking about surgery as a treatment option, make sure you read the entire chapter. Imagine this possibility: you get through your surgery successfully. A few days later, you are one of the fortunate men who receive fantastic news on your post-surgery pathology report. Your cancer was confined to your prostate. You are now cancer free! For a few weeks you are overjoyed at your good fortune.

After a few days or weeks, all the relief and joy has faded from your memory. Now you find yourself so depressed you have fleeting thoughts about taking your own life or wish you'd never treated your cancer at all. In fact, you think you'd have been better off dying from prostate cancer than living the life you have after surgery. You come to the conclusion that choosing surgery was one of the worst decisions you've made in your life.

Emotionally, it gets worse. In addition to being depressed,

you could judge yourself harshly, since you are no longer grateful you've been cured of cancer. Then it's highly likely you will make another decision that will further increase your emotional suffering. You decide to keep these thoughts to yourself. You are certain if you share them with your healthy friends and family, they will tell you not to feel that way, or tell you to feel grateful to be alive. When you hate the quality of your life, being told you should feel grateful is not in the least bit helpful. Your concern about how friends and family would react is probably accurate.

It may be a relief to know that many men with prostate cancer have those feelings. It's not a matter of being ungrateful or crazy. Men do not realize what erections mean to our sense of well-being and manhood until we lose the ability to have one. The majority of men whose nerve bundles were spared will lose the ability to have an erection for eighteen to twenty-four months. During that time, nothing you or your partner can do will give you an erection. Even with ED medication, you are impotent.

Adding insult to injury, at the same time, you are dealing with the loss of urinary control. These two losses devastate your emotional well being and your sense of being a man. Within a few short weeks or months following surgery, you are at risk for a major depression.

Here are some behavioral signs you are experiencing depression:

- ✓ A change in sleep patterns—sleeping more or having difficulty getting to sleep or staying asleep.

- ✓ The loss of the ability to enjoy activities that brought you great pleasure—hobbies, interests, sex, etc.

- ✓ A change in energy level. This can go in two directions—a loss of energy so you become lethargic or you become agitated, making it difficult to sit still.

✓ You become withdrawn and isolate yourself from friends and family.

✓ You lose the ability to laugh.

✓ You have a pervasive negative mood. You may become easily angered or irritated.

✓ You are pessimistic about the quality of your life not only in the present but for the future.

✓ You experience a change in appetite; you lose or gain weight due to a change in eating patterns.

✓ You find yourself unable to complete tasks of daily living such as getting dressed, or working.

✓ You have a significant drop in confidence and self-esteem. Much of the way you think about yourself is in harsh and critical terms.

✓ You find yourself wishing you never had the surgery and think you would have been better off dying of cancer, or you have thoughts of killing yourself.

If you are experiencing depression, it's important for you to do two things. First, it is vital for you to find someone on your team who can hear and understand your pain. It may be necessary for you to join a prostate cancer support group that meets face to face or online. I highly recommend taking this step. The support I received online from other men going through this was incredibly helpful. This support didn't help me avoid depression, they helped me work through it.

The second step would be to consider speaking with your doctor about medication to treat depression. This would be an important step to take if you were depressed prior to your diagnosis of prostate cancer or if there is a family history of depression. Obtaining a psychiatric consultation for the medical management of depression is something else to consider.

It's often difficult to make a clinical distinction between

profound sadness and grief from a depressive episode. In the beginning, sadness, grief, and loss may appear to have the same symptoms as depression. Sad people have the ability to move past their sadness to enjoy some aspects of life. They are able to laugh. Not so when you are depressed. Nothing lifts your mood. Your laughter has left the building. Nothing seems funny anymore. The decision to isolate yourself from other people may be a result of depression. However, something else entirely may be driving your isolating behavior.

Whether you are depressed or sad, it's vitally important for you to find ways to share your thoughts with someone on your team. I experienced six very powerful emotions when I coped with the loss of bladder control and erectile dysfunction. These emotions played a key role in my decision to isolate myself from my wife, friends, family, and outside support. They can also prevent you from seeking outside help. Each of the emotions on this list contributed to my depression.

Here's my list. It's not all-inclusive. You may need to add some of your own emotions to this list or cross some out because some of these may not apply to you. Each and every one of these emotions is so powerful that the presence of one these emotions will have a negative impact on your sense of well-being and mood. Dealing with all of them at once is emotionally overwhelming. There is no quick fix to working through these emotions. Time does not heal all wounds. It's the work you do over the course of time that results in healing.

These are the six emotions I struggled with:

1. Shame

2. Embarrassment

3. Humiliation

4. Disgust

5. Helplessness

6. Despair

Shame is a powerful emotion. Its presence can be debilitating. Shame has nothing to do with what you've done; that's guilt. Shame has to do with who you are. Shame is present when you've passed judgment on yourself and found yourself to be worthless and flawed in such a way that you have no value. There is no redemption possible when you are coping with unhealthy shame.

To heal from shame, you must confront the conclusion you've come to about yourself being hopelessly useless. If you've isolated yourself from your partner, and your marriage is currently stressed or characterized by fighting, this will feed your shame and make it grow. The loss of urinary control and the inability to achieve an erection also feed your shame and increase the intensity of this painful emotion.

Another necessary step toward healing from shame is making a decision to come out of hiding. You need to find a safe place to talk about your shame. It's important to find the right person or persons to talk about your feelings of shame with. Be selective and choose wisely; many people do not have the skills to deal with your feelings of shame in a constructive way.

If you are overwhelmed by shame, I want to encourage you. First, I want you to know you are not alone. Almost every man who's gone through prostate surgery has dealt with the loss of urinary control. It was traumatic each time I'd look in the mirror and saw a man wearing an adult diaper staring back at me. My self-image plummeted to a low I'd never experienced before. It took me a while to realize I could take control of this situation. I needed to learn how to manage and live with diapers and pads so I could get out of the house without leaking through and wetting my pants.

I also felt a profound sense of shame when I could not obtain an erection no matter how excited I felt sexually. In addition, I found it next to impossible to get excited when I was leaking urine nonstop twenty-four/seven. As a couple, we needed to find ways I could bring pleasure to my wife and receive pleasure from her. It was also necessary to find ways to make accommodations for my constant urine leaks. This task was challenging because of the shame I felt. When I was controlled by the powerful emotion of shame, my preference was to withdraw from my wife and avoid sex completely. Unfortunately, choosing that option fed and increased the power of my shame. In order to achieve victory over shame, it's essential to come out of hiding.

It's difficult and embarrassing to work together as a couple to find new ways to experience the joy of satisfying sex. Coming out of hiding means you find people who can help you challenge, confront, and defeat the sources of your shame. Shame is so powerful that it's next to impossible to defeat it alone.

There is no better place to find the necessary support and help to defeat shame than finding couples who've been there and done that. You find those men and women in prostate cancer support groups. Based on your comfort level and availability, you can find a group that meets in person, or you can find support groups online. It's also incredibly valuable to speak with men a little further along than you on the path toward healing. For wives, I give the same advice. Your husband may not buy into the idea of getting support in any way. That shouldn't stop you from finding support. You need as much support as you can get.

Embarrassment is another painful emotion. Embarrassment comes when you experience an event or feeling you want to remain private that becomes public. It's also possible to experience this painful emotion even though an event or feeling remains private. A personal example was wearing diapers in public places. No one knew I was wearing a diaper, but I remember shopping one day and feeling terribly self-conscious. I imagined I was the only person in that store wearing an adult diaper, and this thought bothered me a great deal. This form of embarrassment was generated totally within my mind.

Another form of embarrassment occurs when something goes terribly wrong in public. I was mortified after I went into a restroom stall to empty my small leg bag of urine, which I described earlier. When I missed the toilet, I spilled urine all over my pants. I knew I'd have to pull up my pants, leave the bathroom, and walk through a busy public shopping center with urine-soaked jeans. Finally, I had to make my way through a public parking lot as well. Anyone who looked my way couldn't help but notice my pants. Even though I was not subjected to public ridicule, my sense of embarrassment was sky high.

Sometimes your embarrassment comes from the way you talk to yourself. The way through that type of embarrassment is to challenge and change your internal dialogue. I'll use the example above to illustrate this point. At the mall, I imagined everyone who passed me noticed my urine-soaked pants and was enjoying a good private laugh at my expense. With that attitude, I was so ashamed and embarrassed I wanted to stay in the stall until my pants dried, even if it meant being in there for hours.

Once I left the bathroom, I realized I could either give in to this embarrassment or talk to myself differently. The reality was very few people, perhaps not one, noticed my wet pants. If they did, it was much more likely they'd think I spilled a soft drink on myself. What were the odds someone would think, *Oh, there's an old man who just soaked his pants with urine. That's hilarious.* Once I realized I was not on public display and that anyone who noticed my wet pants would think I spilled a drink on myself, I made it to the car with my head held high. My embarrassment was dramatically reduced when I changed my thinking. I stopped thinking urinary incontinence and erectile dysfunction had stolen my manhood and ruined my life.

I began thinking of urinary incontinence and erectile dysfunction as war injuries. Like any war injury, they required treatment and rehabilitation. The treatment for urinary incontinence was Kegels. The treatment for erectile dysfunction was penile rehabilitation. Wearing black nylon pants, changing my diaper every hour, and carrying a spare set of clothing in a backpack gave me the confidence I needed to venture out in public.

Humiliation involves being brought down to a lower state or status. This may occur from an outside source in the form of ridicule, scorn, criticism, or some other type of public putdown. This painful feeling can also arise based on the way we talk to ourselves. Shortly after I arrived home from the hospital, I was sitting in a reclining chair. I noticed my pants were wet. When I stood up, I noticed I'd wet the chair with urine as well. No one was there to tease me or laugh at me, but I experienced humiliation just the same. I was surprised that my dog, Teddy, helped me put things in the right perspective. Teddy began circling, wagging his tail, and attempting to jump up to get a good sniff at the urine-soaked chair.

Teddy is not housebroken. If he's not let out, he often goes into the downstairs bathroom and urinates by the toilet. It was clear to me Teddy was, in his own way, delighted to discover by his sense of smell he wasn't the only one who urinates in the house. His reaction to this event gave me a welcome, hardy laugh. The power of my humiliation was broken by my laughter.

There was another area where I experienced painful humiliation. This occurred when I could not respond to sexual excitement with an erection. My wife and I agreed it was important to find ways for us to experience orgasms without my having an erection. Most men, myself included, believe you must have an erection in order to experience an orgasm. This isn't true. You can have an enjoyable orgasm with a flaccid penis. It took me a while before I could enjoy this experience because I was mourning the loss of my pre-surgery sex life. However, once we found other ways to receive and give sexual pleasure, my sense of manhood was restored, and the powerful effects of humiliation were defeated.

Disgust is a strong feeling of aversion toward something. It's possible to modify or change your attitudes so things that were disgusting to you no longer elicit this emotion. In the early stages post-surgery, I felt disgusted with everything associated with my sexuality. I would leak urine during foreplay. I'd leak urine when I got excited. Worst of all, I would leak a lot of urine during my orgasm. In fact, it was more like I was urinating rather than leaking. I was totally disgusted by this problem. You tend to avoid things that disgust you, so I avoided sex.

My wife was not disgusted when I leaked urine. Through her accepting eyes, my attitude over time changed as well. I will never like leaking urine during every phase of our sexual relationship. Fortunately, I'm no longer disgusted by it. This means I don't need to avoid sex in order to avoid feeling that painful emotion of disgust. Something else had to change in addition to my attitude. We had to find practical ways to accommodate my leaking urine. At nineteen months post-surgery, we still use a mattress protector. It's also necessary to keep some towels around. As a result of my wife's accepting attitude, the mattress protector, and a few towels, we've made the necessary accommodations for me to relax and enjoy my sexuality.

Helplessness is the belief you have no control or ability to bring about change in the circumstances you are facing. Sometimes there are events that occur beyond our influence or control, so the feeling of helplessness is accurate. For example, no matter how diligently you've been taking care of your health, there was nothing you could have done to prevent your prostate cancer. There are other situations when we mistakenly feel helpless. In those instances, there are actions we can take that can make a difference, but we act as though there isn't anything we can do. For example, for the first two months post-surgery, I was unable to walk ten feet from the toilet to the bath without leaking. I felt helpless with regard to controlling the flow of my urine. I also felt helpless when there was no level of sexual stimuli or ED medication that would give me an erection. With both of those situations, I felt helpless.

When I've driven on a cross-country trip from California to New York, I don't arrive in New York on the first day. At the end of the first day of driving, I don't sit around feeling depressed because I'm not in New York. Additionally, I don't feel helpless even though I'm still thousands of miles from New York because I know I'm measurably closer to New York at the end of the first day. I didn't realize until I regained urinary control that I wasn't helpless. When I did my Kegels every day, I was doing something about my loss of urinary control. Unfortunately, unlike the cross-country drive, I had nothing to show for my effort. At the end of the day, week, or month, I found myself going through the same number of pads. I took this to mean nothing I did mattered and I was not making any progress. This belief was inaccurate.

What I didn't understand at the time is that progress when dealing with urinary incontinence must be measured in a different way. I didn't understand my journey toward urinary control would come at a snail's pace rather than at highway speeds. For some men it will take months before they will experience measurable progress. I tried and failed to alter this fact. My faulty reasoning went like this: if six sets of ten Kegels can heal you in three months, doing twelve sets of ten Kegels a day would cut my recovery time in half.

Rather than helping me heal faster, overdoing the number of Kegels made things significantly worse. Within twenty-four hours of putting this plan into effect, my leaking got worse. It took me a while to understand that by performing too many Kegels, I'd fatigued my sphincter. Something much worse happened as well and quickly put an end to my foolish attempt to speed up my recovery.

I began to experience extremely painful bladder spasms while I was doing my Kegels. I became discouraged when I realized there was nothing I could do to cut my healing time in half. I got so discouraged I stopped doing Kegels completely. I went from one extreme of doing too many to the other extreme of doing none in the span of a week.

It took me a while to challenge my belief that I was helpless. Eventually I realized I needed to continue performing Kegels on a daily basis. Additionally, I learned to trust that I was on the path toward healing, but the pace was not one I could measure day by day.

Another area in which I felt helpless was dealing with impotence. At first I did nothing. I experienced depression and despair. Once I discovered I could not obtain an erection, I tried the vacuum pump. That didn't work well for me. Then I tried ED medication, hoping I would respond. I didn't. Then I decided to combine using the pump with ED medication. I still didn't obtain a useable erection. I came to the conclusion there was nothing I could do but wait eighteen to twenty-four months until my nerve bundles healed from surgery. I felt totally helpless.

Eventually, as I mentioned earlier, I learned it was possible to enjoy orgasms without an erection. I also learned about penile rehabilitation. I decided it was important to resume sexual relations with my wife, so I learned how to perform penile injections. My wife and I were able to resume sexual relations even though I was totally impotent. Once again I'd wrongly assumed I was helpless with regard to erectile dysfunction. When you are overwhelmed by helplessness, feelings of despair aren't far away.

Despair: At some point after surgery, I decided my life was forever ruined. Once you've reached that point, it's easy to believe it would have been better for you to have enjoyed whatever years you had and then die from prostate cancer rather than live with the diminished quality of your life. As I looked to the future, I was devoid of all hope things would ever get better. Once I took the lesson I learned from Charlie Brown and began hating one day at a time rather than hating the entire future, my level of despair dramatically decreased.

Another important way to defeat despair is to find things to celebrate. If you are feeling despair, reread Chapter 8- "Celebrate" before you put the book down for the day. In order to celebrate anything, it means you are looking for positive events in your life to celebrate. Looking for positive developments to celebrate will uplift your outlook on life. The final antidote against despair is instilling hope into your life.

Hope is an expectation that something good will come from your experiences. You believe either the quality of your life will get better or you will find positive ways to cope with your current circumstances. Living without hope will cause you much distress. The Bible gives us some things to hope for so we can have hope right now without our circumstances changing. This is where faith comes in to make a supernatural difference. Psalm 31:24 says, "Be of good courage, and He shall strengthen your heart, all you who hope in the LORD."

Without your circumstances changing or the quality of your life improving, the Bible tells us that once you've made a decision to hope in the Lord, God Himself will strengthen your heart. I can say from personal experience this happened to me. God's help is also available to you. I want you to have realistic expectations. For a while, these powerful negative emotions may win the battle and cause you much emotional distress. With my faith intact, with outside support in place and a loving and supportive wife, there were times during my fifteen diapers a day life that I felt all these powerful emotions.

I also suffered from buyer's remorse. I thought surgery had ruined my life beyond repair. I avoided physical contact with my wife because each touch reminded me of what I had lost and overwhelmed me with grief. I lost my ability to laugh. What I'm saying here is this: there is a season following surgery that can be characterized by a pervasive sense of negativity. Great faith cannot and will not sugar coat your reality or make painful losses not painful. In fact, the Bible says in Ecclesiastes 3:1, "To everything there is a season, a time for every purpose under heaven." There are a few seasons that are essential for you to go through in order to get to the other side of embracing post-surgery life.

Ecclesiastes 3:4 says, "A time to weep." We weep when we feel profound sorrow. Tears must flow in order to keep our humanity intact. There is a season to cry over things that are lost. There's a time when we can bring complaints to God, cry out, and experience the full intensity of feelings of your difficulties adjusting to your life post-surgery.

Ecclesiastes also says, "And a time to laugh." The ability to laugh is in itself healing. It is extremely important for you to find things that are humorous and enjoy them. If you lose the ability to laugh for an extended period of time, it's likely you are suffering from depression.

"A time to mourn." It's important to acknowledge those things that are forever changed and/or lost and work through our feelings about those losses. It took me eight months to mourn the loss of the pleasurable experience of ejaculation. Mourning takes time.

"And a time to dance." There's a time for celebration. Usually we don't dance alone. Dancing involves a partner. It's important to find ways to celebrate with other people.

"And a time to heal." My favorite seasons of healing occur when there is a complete restoration of things that were lost. Healing also occurs when we've said good-bye to that which is lost to us forever and are able to embrace what we have left. On this journey we can experience healing physically, emotionally, relationally, and spiritually.

To experience healing in these areas, it requires intentionally on our part.

Moving through seasons takes time and effort. Here are a just a few factors that influence how you and your partner will cope with each season:

- ❏ Your experiences in your family of origin
- ❏ Your personality style
- ❏ Your degree of emotional maturity
- ❏ Your history of coping as a couple
- ❏ Your faith
- ❏ Other stresses in your life

Grieving together is a difficult endeavor. Each person grieves differently. The time it takes for each of you to move through a season of grief will vary. It is also possible different coping styles can stretch your relationship to the breaking point. If this happens, I hope you would place a higher value on your marriage than your pride or shame. Both of these feelings can prevent you from seeking out help during extremely stressful seasons of your life.

Men, listen up. If your wife says your marriage is in trouble, believe her. If you ignore your wife as she gives you this warning, things will get worse and your marriage could end. Withdrawing and ignoring problems make things worse, not better.

Here's a word picture to help you understand what I'm saying. Imagine your home is on fire. You are in another room far away from the fire. There is no way you can feel the heat or see the fire with your own eyes. You are the one who is by the only phone in the house. In order to prevent your house from burning down, you'll need to trust your wife's warning to pick up the phone and call the fire department. If you trusted your wife's warning, help came and your home was saved. If you ignored your wife's warning, your house burned to the ground. It's like that with your marriage. If your wife says your relationship is in trouble, you need to hear and believe her. If you choose to ignore your wife's warning, then you are as foolish as the man who wouldn't call the fire department. The damage you refuse to deal with can destroy your relationship in the season you need a helpmate the most.

You may feel entirely worthless and defective as a man and be convinced your wife would be better off without you. It's possible you will behave in such a way as to drive your wife away because you believe that's what you deserve. Think back to your wedding vows. There was a reason you pledged to stay together in sickness and in health. God intends for your marriage to be a place where you help one another through all of life's trials. One of those trials is prostate cancer. Now more than ever you need to find ways to become helpmates to one another.

Questions/Thoughts for Discussion

1. Take time to write down the seasons you've been through and the season you are in right now.

2. Share your seasons with each other. Talk about where you've been and where you are today.

3. What did you learn about yourself, your partner, and your marriage?

4. Are either of you stuck in a painful season? If so, what season, and what is needed to help get through it?

5. Do you need outside support for you as an individual?

6. Do you need outside support to help your relationship? If so, will you do this as a couple?

7. If you are refusing to seek help when your helpmate says it's necessary, what's preventing you from seeking help together?

8. If one of you must go for help alone, describe how that decision will change your relationship.

Chapter 28

What in the World Is Penile Rehab?

If you are one of the fortunate men who quickly regains his erectile abilities, then penile rehab is unnecessary for you. I have no idea how or why I expected a return of my erectile functioning within three months after surgery. Based on my incorrect assumption, I saw no reason to read and prepare myself for something I was certain I wouldn't need.

Three months post-surgery all my attempts to achieve an erection with ED medication failed. In *Saving Your Sex Life*, Dr. John Mulhall, states the majority of men will not respond to medication immediately following surgery. It takes between eighteen and twenty-four months, sometimes longer, for men before they regain erectile abilities. To say that finding myself in this group was a major disappointment would be an understatement. I was closer to being devastated.

How couples feel and cope with the months or years without intercourse is varied. For some couples, it is not a big deal. For some men, the idea of living without intercourse is so traumatic they'd rather die of prostate cancer than face a few months or years, of impotence. A healthier way to reframe this sentiment is: for some men, the potential risks involved with surgery are too high. Finding another way to treat prostate cancer is necessary.

Once I was diagnosed with prostate cancer, I noticed my sex drive (often referred to as "libido") was dramatically reduced. Coping with urinary incontinence after surgery reduced it even further. The fact that I couldn't stop leaking urine made the whole idea of sex repulsive. At that point, I had no interest in sex, nor did I care whether I regained my erectile function. Frankly, I was amazed my wife was more concerned about my being proactive about penile rehab than I was. For the first few months following surgery, I didn't care when or if my nerve bundles healed.

In direct contrast to my passivity, my wife was a woman on a mission. She wanted me to do everything in my power to restore my erectile abilities. I started penile rehab reluctantly and more to please my wife than out of my own desire. I was fortunate to find a lecture on this topic on YouTube.[2] Every man who is thinking about surgery should listen to Dr. Mulhall's lecture about penile rehab. It's amazing we live in the information age, yet so many men who choose surgery receive little or no information about this important topic.

After listening to his lecture, I bought Dr. Mulhall's book, appropriately titled *Saving Your Sex Life: A Guide for Men with Prostate Cancer.* Dr. Mulhall writes about a serious and potentially avoidable condition that riveted my attention. It's called "venous leak."

An erection is produced when blood to the penis compresses the veins in the corpora cavernosa so the blood cannot leave. Venous leakage occurs when these veins do not close enough to retain the blood. This means you cannot maintain a useable erection. This condition does not heal. Once you develop a venous leak you will

---

2 http://www.youtube.com/watch?v=ie8NkOu2VNA, accessed April 2012.

not have another erection without corrective surgery or a penile implant.

According to Dr. Mulhall, if men do not get a blood flow into the penis on a regular basis following surgery, the risk for developing venous leak increases. In fact, the longer a man goes without a regular blood flow, the higher the risk for developing a venous leak. No one warned me of this possibility prior to surgery. Once I understood the consequences of a venous leak, I became as frightened of developing a venous leak as I was with the diagnosis of prostate cancer.

Additionally, as many as half the men who have nerve-sparing surgery will develop a venous leak within twelve months. I did not want to be one of those men! However, when I learned how Dr. Mulhall treats men who are not responsive to ED medication, I found myself ready to give up on the idea of penile rehab. For men like me who had no response to ED medication, his recommended course of treatment is penile injections. I'd never heard of penile injections, nor would I ever consider sticking a needle into my penis.

My son Andy often quotes a phrase he learned from a cartoon he watched as a child: "When in doubt, take the easy way out." That's exactly what I intended to do. I was determined to find an alternative way of getting a blood flow into my penis.

When you take the easy way out, you make sacrifices. Unfortunately, a vacuum pump does not bring highly oxygenated blood to the penis. According to Dr. Mulhall, there's no concrete evidence a pump preserves penile tissue. However, I figured a little oxygenated blood was better than no oxygenated blood. On the next post-surgical visit to UCSF, I asked for a prescription for a vacuum pump. I had two goals. The first was to use the pump to help get a blood flow into my penis. My second was to use the pump to obtain an erection in order to resume sexual relations with my wife.

Once I got the pump home, I tried using it. On a zero-to-ten scale, with zero meaning no erection and a ten a full erection, I discovered that even if I pumped myself until the batteries were drained of power, I couldn't get past a level five of hardness. I knew what to do next. I decided to take ED medication prior to using the pump. I was certain this combination would give me a useable erection. It didn't. Additionally, getting the ring to fit properly was another challenge. If you don't get the ring directly on the base of the penis, you will be flaccid behind the ring and hard in front of it.

I tried using the combination of ED meds with the vacuum pump three times a week for almost a month without obtaining a useable erection. I was now almost four months post-surgery without a useable erection. The specter of developing a venous leak loomed in my mind. There were no good solutions. I could either wait the eighteen to twenty-four months for my nerve bundles to heal and risk the possibility of developing a venous leak, or I could go back to UCSF and learn how to perform penile injections. I seriously hated both options. In the end, I found my fear of developing a venous leak was greater than my fear of penile injections.

Within the week, I called UCSF to learn everything I never wanted to learn about penile injections. They cautiously started me off with a low dose of Bi-mix since I'd had an episode of priapism (an erection lasting four hours) while taking Flomax. After my nurse showed me where to inject, I was unpleasantly surprised she handed me the needle. It was obvious she expected me to perform the injection. I took the needle and successfully performed my first penile injection. Afterwards, the nurse closed the curtain around the exam table. She said she was leaving the room so I could stimulate myself to see whether I would obtain an erection. I thought she was kidding.

I was sitting with my pants down to my ankles and my heart pounding, recovering emotionally from giving myself a penile injection. I couldn't imagine a single sexual thought that would excite me. My levels of anxiety and embarrassment were too high, and my imagination wasn't that good. The nurse returned in ten minutes. She felt the base of my penis and said it was engorged and that was a good sign. I didn't share her optimism. I'd only achieved a hardness level of two or three which was nowhere close to being hard enough to achieve penetration. I considered the results an abysmal failure, so I asked her why she was pleased.

She said based on the level of engorgement, it was clear Bi-mix would work for me. The only issue was to find the correct dosage. I stayed in the examination room forty-five minutes. I was mildly engorged the entire time. This meant I did not have a venous leak. This was wonderful news. Then she said something that would help me get through some difficult times injecting—that penile injecting would speed up the recovery time of my nerve bundles. This gave me a sense of having some control over the course of my healing. At four months post-surgery I hadn't experienced an erection. I drove home feeling grateful because the long wait for an erection was about to end.

Finding the right dosage is a process that cannot be hurried. It's important to move slowly or you could end up in the emergency room with an erection that won't go down. If an erection lasts more than four hours, it is a medical emergency. Without intervention, you could experience permanent penile tissue damage.

As much as I wanted to find the right dose as quickly as possible, I followed the instructions to the letter. I was told to increase the dosage by small increments until I was able to achieve erection hardness between seven and eight that would last forty-five minutes to an hour. By the third injection, I found the correct dosage.

Once I found the correct dosage, I was pleased to experience a useable erection. I was delighted my wife and I were able to resume sexual relations. Unfortunately, this wasn't a happily-ever-after experience. Injecting a needle into your penis takes some getting used to. Oddly, I discovered I did not gain confidence regarding my skills with injecting as time went on. Instead, I became increasingly fearful. My worst fears were realized on my fifth injection.

I did the usual search, making sure I wouldn't inject into a vein. As I pushed the needle into my penis, I wanted more than anything simply to pull it out and quit. Somehow I managed to keep pushing until the needle was all the way in. Slowly I expelled the medication, pulled out the needle, and compressed the injection site. I knew what was coming next—ten to fifteen seconds of a burning sensation. I wasn't disappointed. I groaned in agony, and then the pain left. I breathed a sigh of relief; I'd successfully completed injection number five.

My relief was short-lived. I happened to glance at the palm of my left hand. It was bloody. I knew I wasn't bleeding at the injection site because the pad I was using to apply compression was white, not red. Blood was flowing out of my urethra. I grabbed some toilet paper and began wiping up the flowing blood. My wife suggested I lie down and compress the area. I followed her suggestion, and the bleeding stopped within a few minutes.

I was convinced I'd injected in the wrong area, which meant I would not have an erection. I was ticked off and turned off. I was ticked off because I'd just experienced the pain of the injection and endured the painful burning, and after all that I still wouldn't have an erection. I was turned off because I was seriously traumatized to see blood flowing out of my penis. I doubted I would ever want to inject a needle into my penis again.

I was also feeling sorry for myself because of the changes the prostate surgery had brought to my sex life. While lying in bed compressing my penis to stop the bleeding, I held a pity party for myself. I was the guest of honor. As the pity party got into full swing, I looked down and was shocked and surprised to discover I had an erection, even though I hadn't entertained a single sexual thought. After all that emotional and physical suffering, I wasn't about to waste a useable erection, so my wife and I enjoyed our time together.

We were both delighted we could share an intimate experience together. A short time later I was surprised when I found myself feeling strangely alienated and disconnected from my body. I realized no amount of pleasure could excite me to the point of getting an erection. From the other direction, once I injected correctly, it seemed no amount of pain or disgust prevented me from obtaining an erection. I lost total control of my sexual responsiveness. I felt like a mechanical man, dependent on a needle in order to achieve an erection.

To make matters worse, after the episode of blood flowing out of my urethra, I became terrified of injecting. Quitting was an appealing option. My second option was to push through the fear and try injecting again the next week. Since I had no idea what I had done wrong or how to prevent the bleeding from occurring a second time, I rejected the idea of trying again, hoping for a different outcome. I was stuck (pun intended). Neither option appealed to me.

My wife suggested I call UCSF and speak to the nurse who taught me how to inject. At first I rejected the idea. I was way too embarrassed to admit I made a mistake injecting. However, this was the only way I'd get the information I needed. It took me three days to come to a decision. A Bible verse guided my choice, from (2 Timothy 1:7): "For God has not given us a spirit of fear but of power and of love and of a sound mind."

Getting help wasn't as easy as it sounds. On day one I called UCSF. I had to tell the person on the phone why I needed to speak with the nurse practitioner who taught me how to inject. That was difficult, but I did it. I received a call back on my cell phone at 6:30 p.m. Since I was eating, I missed the call. The nurse left a message telling me how to deal with the issue of blood in my urine after I injected. She told me I'd be okay and that I should drink plenty of fluids.

Seeing blood in my urine after injecting was not the problem. The advice I was given was not for the problem I'd experienced. I knew I'd have to call UCSF a second time and had to face my embarrassment again. It also meant I'd have to tell another person what had happened. The next day I called UCSF. I explained this was my second phone call and it was important I speak directly to the nurse practitioner who had taught me how to inject. I was put on hold and then told she was doing a procedure. They assured me I would receive a call back once the procedure was finished. I did not receive a call back that day.

On day three, I called UCSF again. By now I was no longer embarrassed. Frustration replaced embarrassment, and anger was beginning to surface. Most urologists' offices are extremely busy. Getting help for a non-medical emergency takes time, patience, and persistence. It would have been convenient to use these delays as an excuse to quit injecting. Some men are not assertive by nature. They will give up after one or two failed attempts to get help. I want to encourage any man who becomes quickly discouraged to get the support you need to help you do what you need to do rather than to quit.

Beside the temptation to quit, there is another temptation. It's a strong one. I've given in to this one too many times in other circumstances. It's the strategy to use anger to resolve a problem. By day three, I could have easily justified the idea of screaming at the staff for neglecting my request for help twice. If you are one of those men who frequently uses anger, threats, or intimidation to resolve problems, you will find yourself acting harshly to the very people who you want and need to take care of you. That's not a particularly wise strategy. Proverbs 21:23 says, "Whoever guards his mouth and tongue keeps his soul from troubles." I strongly advise you to demonstrate kindness to the people whose help you need. Dumping anger on them does more damage than good.

On my third phone call, my persistence paid off. I explained the problem and informed her this was my third phone call to resolve this issue. I was put on hold, and the next person who came to the phone was my nurse practitioner. I explained what had happened. She was great. She listened to what had happened and told me I'd probably injected too low and punctured my urethra with the needle. If you think of the top of your penis as 12:00, it's safe to inject at 2:00 and 10:00 or 3:00 or 9:00.

Apparently, I was so focused on missing my veins that I neglected to watch where I placed the needle. I ended up injecting at 6:00. From that position, I hit my urethra. I discovered as I rehearsed for my next injection that I lose my orientation when I pull, stretch, and turn my penis for the injection. I decided I'd need to mark the injection site so I wouldn't make the same mistake a second time. For every injection from that day on, I'd use a marker and then draw a small circle on my penis indicating where to inject. I'd use an alcohol pad to sterilize the area inside the circle, making sure I didn't wipe away the circle.

With this technique, I was certain I'd never make that mistake a second time. I was finally developing a sense of confidence and competence in performing penile injections. It was unbelievable that I lost my newly found competence after the very next injection. I did everything right. I found the correct site and stuck the needle in. I felt the familiar pain after pushing in the Bi-mix. Afterward I compressed the area. I let out a sigh of relief because everything went perfectly. I joined my wife in bed. For the first time since I began injecting with the correct dosage, I remained flaccid.

I became angry, frustrated, and confused. Previously, when I did everything wrong and had blood flowing out of my penis, I obtained an erection. This time, I did everything right. I was in the mood, ready, and willing, but

I was unable to obtain an erection after my injection. (Cool rhyme, wasn't it?)

The following week I tried again. I experienced the same frustrating failure. My injection statistics were now zero for two. I felt ready and justified to give up on penile injections. I certainly understand why the dropout rate in the first three months of injecting is so high. I wanted to be one of those men who quit during the first three months. However, I asked myself a single question, which ruled out the option for quitting: *If I quit, am I willing to risk the possibility of developing a venous leak and permanently losing the ability to have an erection?* The answer was a resounding no. In fact, rather than waiting a week, I decided I needed to try injecting again the very next day. It was the first and only time I was willing to inject twice in the same week.

I achieved an erection barely hard enough for penetration. I didn't understand what was going wrong. I'd found a dose where I'd achieved a strong erection that lasted forty-five minutes. With that same dose, I'd failed completely twice. The third time, I achieved a barely useable erection that lasted a few minutes. I went totally flaccid before either of us could achieve an orgasm.

Fortunately, we took a two-week vacation out of state with our daughter. The timing of that vacation was perfect. I needed a break. Once we returned from our vacation, I began injecting again. Thankfully, with the increased dose/ dosage, I was able to obtain a good erection. However, something else happened that made me want to quit. Rather than acclimating to the pain of inserting a needle into my penis, I found it was becoming increasingly more difficult. I'd start to push the needle in, feel the pain, and pull the needle out.

It reached a crisis point when I had to poke myself three times before I got the needle embedded for an injection. What was happening was confusing and counterintuitive. When I first learned how to inject, I had no difficulty using the right amount of pressure to get the needle fully embedded into my penis. For reasons I cannot explain, over the course of time, putting a needle into my penis became increasingly difficult rather than easier.

I know men who decided they wanted penile injections but didn't want to be the one to perform them. They had their partners go to the training session and learn the technique. Even though my wife is an RN, I did not want Brenda involved in the process of performing my penile injections. I considered the process of injecting extremely anti-romantic. I didn't want to involve her with this mood killing experience.

Within three months of injecting, I'd hit a wall. I did not want my wife to give me my injections, nor did I want to stick another needle into my penis. I found myself unwilling to inject, but I did not want to quit. My first conversation regarding the possibility of using an auto injector occurred when I ordered my first prescription of Bi-mix. The pharmacist told me he received so many complaints from men who purchased auto injectors, he stopped selling them. He advised me not to waste my time or money with an auto injector. I heeded his warning.

I became so averse to injecting, I began losing sleep the night before. Any sense of delightful anticipation, joy, or pleasure associated with sex was now replaced with an awful sense of dread. It became evident I was experiencing too much pain emotionally and physically to continue on this path. Since I was ready to quit, I thought I had nothing to lose by trying out the auto injector.

I thought finding one would be easy, but it wasn't. The compounding pharmacy where I purchased my Bi-mix didn't sell them. When I went into a nationally known pharmacy and asked about auto injectors, they didn't carry them either. So I did what I always do to find something—I went to my favorite search engine and typed in the words "auto injector." Immediately I found what I was looking for. If I had called UCSF, I'm sure they would have given me a prescription, and insurance might have covered the expense.

I didn't want to go through that process, so I purchased the injector on my own. I paid approximately thirty-five dollars. It arrived within seven days.

When I opened the box, I wasn't impressed. The injector was all plastic. I was certain if I pulled too hard on the latch, I'd easily break it. The first task was to figure out how to place the needle in the injector and lock it in place. Once that was accomplished, I needed to find the right combination of adapters and rings. The goal was to find the right setting to ensure the needle would be fully exposed once the trigger was pressed. When this was accomplished, I must have pushed the trigger a dozen times trying to anticipate how much pain I'd experience when I put the injector against my penis and pulled the trigger.

The words of my pharmacist, "The majority of men find the auto injector too painful to use," echoed in my mind. I'd already reached a point where self-injecting was too painful. The possibility the auto injector would increase the level of pain was frightening. I thought about testing the auto injector on my thigh, but I stopped myself from carrying out this experiment. I realized if it hurt, I'd throw the auto injector away before using it on my penis. It was important to perform a penile injection with the auto injector in spite of my fears.

After filling the needle with the correct dosage of Bi-mix, I loaded the needle into the injector. I marked the injection site with a marker. I used an alcohol pad to sterilize the area, positioned the injector within the circle, and pushed the trigger. I closed my eyes and braced myself for pain. I was pleasantly surprised. It didn't hurt. In fact, I was so busy thinking about how little pain I'd experienced that I forgot to press the plunger down to release the medication! After a few seconds, the pain of the embedded needle reminded me to push the medication in.

My first experience with auto injecting was painless and quite successful. I was overjoyed. The auto injector brought me from the brink of quitting to feeling confidant

I could continue with penile injections. I may be in the minority of men, but the auto injector became a necessity. I would have quit injecting without one. If you ask your urologist's office for a prescription for the auto injector, it may be covered by your insurance. My suggestion is to try both methods of injecting. Choose the one best suited to your preferences. If the idea of injecting your penis is so intolerable to you, ask your partner if they would learn how give you the injections.

With the auto injector, I found injecting tolerable. I was ready to continue until my nerve bundles healed. When you find the correct dose, you continue to use it. As your nerve bundles begin to heal you'll begin to stay erect longer than forty-five minutes. Once that happens, it's important to gradually decrease your dose of Bi-mix until your nerve bundles are healed. That's what I was told to expect. I wasn't surprised, when the exact opposite happened to me.

Over the span of the next three months, it was taking increasingly larger doses of medication to achieve an erection until the day injecting failed completely. Eventually, I could not obtain an erection with an entire needle full of Bi-mix. At first I thought this meant I had a bad batch of medication. Even though it was still within the expiration date, I called for a refill.

When the new medication arrived, I lowered the dose to the level I used when I had my last successful erection. It didn't work. I gradually increased the dose until I'd pushed a needle full of Bi-mix without obtaining an erection. By now I had injected six times without achieving a single usable erection. I realized it was time to call UCSF again. I spoke with my nurse practitioner. She recommended I come in for a consult. I told her I needed some time to think about it.

I had a list of reasons I didn't want to go back to UCSF to try a different medication:

❖ I'd just spent seventy-five dollars for a new batch of medication that failed. I didn't want to spend another seventy-five dollars on another type of medication.

❖ Tri-mix could also fail.

❖ I didn't want to take a day off from work.

❖ I hate driving one hundred eighty miles for a medical appointment.

❖ I hate injecting in a doctor's office.

❖ I find it humiliating to have the nurse practitioner examine my penis after I inject.

For men with a very high sex drive, the motivation to overcome any and all obstacles is built in. My libido was returning very slowly. It was nowhere near the level it was prior to my diagnosis. The question every man has to ask himself once he begins injecting is whether the pain is worth the pleasure. If that was the only equation, I'd have said no and quit, but a Bible verse came to my mind: "Let nothing be done through selfish ambition or conceit, but in lowliness of mind let each esteem others better than himself. Let each of you look out not only for his own interests, but also for the interests of others" (Philippians 2:3–4).

God made it possible to have everything I needed for Brenda and me to continue our sex life together. She couldn't have been more supportive. There was no way I was going to allow pain or discouragement to lead me to quit injecting. I called UCSF to schedule an appointment. They could see me in six weeks.

As I waited for my appointment, I thought two significant events occurred which were signs my nerve bundles were beginning to heal. I'd been taking half a pill of Levitra a few times a week. One day I took a full pill. After some foreplay, I had an erection hard enough for penetration. This was the first time I'd had a response to ED medication.

A few nights later, I had my first nighttime erection. I was delighted. I came to the conclusion responsiveness to ED medication and my first nighttime erection since surgery were conclusive signs my nerve bundles were healed.

Unfortunately, my conclusion was incorrect. The next time I tried Levitra, I was unable to obtain an erection. My nighttime erection was a one-time event. Injections stopped working. I experienced multiple failures with ED medication, and I weeks went by without another nighttime erection.

My hopes that my nerve bundles were beginning to heal and I was recovering from ED were dashed. In fact, I was worse off now than I was three months earlier when injections were working. I had no idea why, but it was evident to me, my ED got worse, rather than better. I thought desperate times call for desperate measures.

I was about to do something I was told never to do. I decided to combine my ED medication with an injection. I knew I was taking a serious risk of experiencing an episode of priapism. I knew I could end up in the emergency room, but I was too desperate to care. A few hours after taking Levitra, I went into the bathroom and closed the door. I set the needle into the auto injector and pushed the trigger, expecting to feel a brief stab of pain as the needle embedded itself into my penis. Nothing happened. I knew why. It meant the needle was not properly locked in place in the injector.

I seriously wondered if this was a sign to quit injecting. It felt as though I was facing a firing squad. I heard the words, "Ready, aim, fire," only to discover the guns weren't loaded. Now it was time to face the firing squad a second time. I locked the needle into place, positioned the injector firmly into the correct area for injecting, and pushed the trigger a second time. It failed a second time. If it failed a third time, I had every intention of throwing the auto injector in the garbage and telling my wife I was finished with penile injections. A lot was riding on the next push of the trigger.

I pushed the trigger a third time. This time the needle embedded in my penis. Pushing in a full needle of Bi-mix felt like shooting fire into my penis. It took approximately five seconds to push in the entire dose. As soon as I pulled the needle out, I felt an intense urge to urinate. I quickly sat on the toilet so I could be comfortable compressing the injection site while urinating. When I stood up, I was unpleasantly surprised. I began squirting urine on my leg, on my pajamas, and on the rug. Now I had to take off my pajamas, wash my leg, and clean the rug. At that point I asked myself, "Why did this happen?" I remembered. I wanted to have a romantic time with my wife. I asked myself a follow-up question: "How's that working out for you?" "Not so well," I replied.

At a time, when I was hoping for a pleasant sexual experience, I was forcefully reminded of the two most miserable consequences of prostate surgery. The first was the need to inject because I'd lost my ability to have an erection. The second was incomplete bladder control. These were not romantic thoughts to have as I left the bathroom to join my wife in bed.

While lying in bed, I reviewed my overall experiences with injecting. I realized every one of my experiences involved physical pain from the injection or the medication. I was never certain whether I'd achieve an erection. More often than not, I'd experience pain for many hours after I injected. No wonder the idea of sex was losing its appeal. Prior to my prostate cancer, if someone had asked me what word came to mind when I heard the word *sex,* my answer would have been pleasure. Now, after surgery, when I asked myself that question, four new words crossed my mind: needles, blood, urine, and pain, not a little, not brief pain, but a lot of pain for long periods of time.

I knew given my current thinking it would take a miracle to obtain an erection. I guess it was my day for a miracle because I was able to obtain one. Despite the difficult start, my wife and I enjoyed a wonderful and highly pleasurable experience together. I was amazed and grateful this was possible. The experience ended every quickly as once again I became flaccid within minutes.

Four hours later, shooting pain in my penis reminded me it was time for a dose of acetaminophen. Twelve hours after injecting, I still was experiencing pain, which required another dose of acetaminophen. As much as I wanted to enjoy my sexual relationship with my wife, injecting and pain were taking a toll on me.

A week later, I tried once again to obtain an erection with ED medication alone. While my erection didn't last as long as I would have liked, I was definitely having a response. I wondered if I should cancel my appointment with UCSF and give up injecting.

We decided to keep the appointment. At that appointment, I explained that while I had some signs of nerve bundle healing, the Bi-mix had completely stopped working. My nurse practitioner was so puzzled by this that she called to consult with a physician. I felt relief that I wasn't the only one who thought this problem was unusual. Unfortunately, the physician was unavailable, which didn't matter since there was nothing anyone could do to make Bi-mix work for me. My next option was to try Tri-mix. The nurse practitioner prepared the dose and handed it to me to inject. She wanted to evaluate my injection technique to determine whether or not I was injecting correctly.

I put the needle with Tri-mix into in my handy dandy auto injector, I showed her where I was going to inject. I placed the auto injector on my penis, pulled the trigger and pushed through the medication. When I was finished, she told me my placement and technique were both correct. This was unfortunate news to hear. I was hoping the problem I experienced would be easy to explain and resolve, instead it remained a mystery. Now the only thing left to assess was whether Tri-mix would work and produce and erection.

After the injection, I had fifteen minutes behind the

curtain to stimulate myself and imagine exciting sexual scenarios. Once again, I found myself with an imagination deficit. Exciting thoughts were not coming to mind. Instead, I began feeling an intensely painful burning sensation in my penis. After fifteen minutes, the nurse practitioner returned. She was surprised to discover my total lack of response to the Tri-mix. She asked me if I wanted to go home with a prescription for Tri-mix so I could begin increasing the dose to see whether it would work.

The extremely painful burning in my penis from the Tri-mix was not something I was willing to experience a second time. I told her there was no way I'd ever inject another dose of Tri-mix. It was obvious to all of us my days of injecting were over. Before leaving, I asked for acetaminophen to reduce the pain. She gave me 1,000 mg. I was in so much pain, I would have preferred morphine.

My wife and daughter wanted to go shopping in San Francisco after my appointment. As they shopped together, my level of pain was way too high for me to focus on anything other than relieving the burning sensation I felt in my penis. While they shopped in department stores, I searched for a pharmacy. When I found one, I purchased a bottle of acetaminophen. I took another 1,000 mg, hoping for some relief. Forty-five minutes later, I was still in too much pain to consider driving home. I asked my liver to forgive me, and took another 1,000 mg. In less than ninety minutes I downed 3,000mg of acetaminophen. Shortly thereafter my pain level dropped to a tolerable level, and I was able to drive our family home. When we pulled into our driveway, I got out of my car and tossed my auto injector into the garbage pail. My days of injecting had come to an abrupt end. Brenda and I breathed a collective sigh of relief. We were ready to enter the next phase of penile rehabilitation.

I wanted to try different brands of ED medication to see which brand produced the best results with the least number of side effects. The first gave me such a painful migraine headache, I would give up sexual relations before

I'd voluntarily experience another migraine. The second brand gave me severe backaches. It was obvious, I'd have to stay on Levitra. The reactions and side effects to each drug will vary from man to man. If you experience a severe side effect, with one medication, don't quit, try another.

At nineteen months after surgery, useable erections with ED medication are a hit and miss experience. We decided to remove all pressure from our sex life, it only serves to make things worse. Attaining a useable erection is no longer our goal. If it happens that's wonderful, if it doesn't, oh well. Our goal with my on-going penile rehab is to keep blood flowing into my penis a few times a week. Achieving a partial erection that isn't useable is considered a successful penile rehab experience. We will continue to do this until I achieve a reliable response to ED medication.

If my writing could influence my outcome, I would have written my story in this way: I successfully continued with penile injections until my nerve bundles healed. As I look back, I am grateful I conquered my fears and learned how to perform penile injections. I could not and would not sit back, and do nothing for two years other than hope my erectile abilities would return. Despite our many setbacks, we've been highly successful. There are times I attain a useable erection. Every few weeks I'll experience a prolonged nighttime erection. As a result of our perservance with penile rehab, I have not developed a venous leak and my nerve bundles continue to heal.

I am in the group of men who need a minimum of twenty-four months before I can hope to experience reliable erections. Brenda and I have adjusted to this reality and enjoy what we are able to enjoy as we wait expectantly for greater healing over the course of time. It's up to you and your partner to find a rehab program that will work for you. The decisions you make will affect your sexual abilities and your relationship for years to come. If you are interested in preserving your erectile functioning, take penile rehab seriously.

Questions to Consider

1. Did your surgeon discuss the importance of penile rehab with you?

2. What form of rehab do you feel most comfortable with?

3. Do you understand how men develop venous leaks?

4. Are you willing to consider penile injections if you are unresponsive to ED medication? If so, why? If not, why not?

5. What does your partner think of your decision?

Chapter 29

Thoughts and Emotions
That Wound

Many years ago, before I accepted Jesus as my Savior, I worked as a medical social worker in a hospital and years later on a kidney dialysis unit. I'll never forget when a woman with terminal cancer told me she was convinced her cancer came as a punishment from God for something she'd done.

After that experience, I routinely began asking patients with chronic or terminal illness if they thought their illness was a punishment from God. I was surprised at the number of people who expressed this belief. Back then I didn't know who God was, and I was glad I didn't. I wouldn't have lasted a day with an angry God who sends terminal illnesses to punish people for doing things wrong.

I've come to know God. I know Him through His Word, the Bible, and through knowing His Son, Jesus. I know God doesn't allow men to get prostate cancer as a punishment for the sins they committed. If that were true, every man on the planet would have prostate cancer. The Bible is quite clear on this matter. On the cross, Jesus took our punishment for every sin we committed or would commit in our past, present, and future. His death on the cross would become unnecessary and meaningless if God continued to punish us for our sins.

Here's a list of thoughts and emotions that will wound you and make a bad situation worse:

❖ "God gave me this cancer as punishment for something I've done wrong." With this belief, your anger and fear will draw you away from God rather than toward Him.

❖ Self-pity is an unending sense of feeling sorry for yourself in a way that resists all comfort. Self-pity becomes unhealthy when you find yourself alone and either unwilling or unable to leave your pity party. At that point, you may be dealing with a serious depression that will require treatment. If you resist all attempts people are making to reach you and isolate yourself from all positive influences, I urge you to seek out professional help. If you are stuck in a pity party, you will not or cannot go to the places God wants you to go. In addition, you will miss out on the comfort and blessings God has prepared just for you in this time of illness and trouble.

❖ Discouragement is the precursor to quitting. There is a sense of futility, so you say to yourself, *Why bother doing anything? It doesn't make a difference one way or the other.* Here are some thoughts I've had that were discouraging.

  ✓ Living with urinary incontinence is hell. My life is ruined forever. I'm sorry I had the surgery.

  ✓ Without ejaculations, I'll never enjoy sex again.

  ✓ I'll never be able to satisfy my wife; maybe she'd be better off with someone else.

  ✓ I'll never regain my manhood.

✓ I'm all alone. No one could understand what I'm going through.

✓ I must avoid all sexual and physical contact with my partner.

✓ I can't trust anyone.

✓ Prostate cancer ruined my life. There's very little left to enjoy.

✓ My faith isn't making a difference with how I'm coping.

❖ Fear is an unpleasant emotion brought on by a real or imagined threat or danger. We generally react to fear with a desire to fight or flee. Fear is distressing to us. We can lose our ability to concentrate, sleep, and perform tasks.

❖ Losing your perspective by believing the worst. Rather than believing the symptoms you are experiencing, such as erectile dysfunction and the loss of urinary control, are temporary, you think these symptoms are never-ending, causing you to hate your life.

❖ Depression is a pervasive sadness and pessimism about the future. You could experience difficulty getting out of bed or performing tasks of daily living. You will withdraw from relationships and neglect personal care. Men may suffer from an agitated depression. Rather than being lethargic, these men can't seem to stop moving. Rather than feeling a pervasive sense of sadness, they primarily feel anger and agitation. They may pace, have racing thoughts, or be unable to complete tasks because of difficulty focusing. Their primary emotions expressed are anger and irritability.

❖ Anxiety is the experience of an unpleasant and unwelcome emotion due to anticipating negative events related to the diagnosis or treatment of your cancer. Severe anxiety may affect your ability to sleep, your ability to think clearly, and your ability to retain information or perform familiar tasks.

❖ Bitterness comes into our lives when we can't let go of our disappointment, hurt, and anger.

If these or other negative emotions are prevalent in your life for a few consecutive months, I believe it would be helpful for you to seek outside help. Living through the everyday realities following prostate surgery is difficult. Being weighed down by thoughts that wound is like trying to tread in water with fifty-pound weights attached to each leg. Eventually you will sink. There is no shame in seeking help. It is the wise thing to do. It's the manly thing to do. By now I sound like a broken record. I've purposely repeated multiple times this idea of seeking help because of how difficult a decision it is to make. Our tendency is to bear emotional and relational suffering alone, rather than seek help.

An example of this occurs when you are lost, and you refuse to stop to get directions. As a consequence of that choice, you'll spend valuable time going in the wrong direction. It takes longer to get to your destination. This is true in our marriages as well. The difficult emotional and physical issues cause us to lose our way. There are places God wants to take you in your marriage, and without the necessary help, you'll remain stuck. There is so much at stake, and it's possible you are too angry or depressed to care.

Some people have a strong need to control every aspect of their lives. They live with a false belief they are in control of their lives and their destiny. Prostate cancer shatters that illusion. When you lose an important belief or way of coping with the world, it's natural to become fearful or angry. In this state, we can maintain the ability to be polite to strangers while we heap anger on those who love us the most. Rather than working through the hurt and releasing it, we feed it. We nurture it. We relive it over and over again many times a day. Each time we relive it, another layer of anger and resentment builds. You can't recover emotionally if you are stuck with repetitive thoughts that wound.

Questions to Consider

1. What thoughts that wound do you experience?

2. How have those wounding thoughts affected your most important relationships with:

   Your partner

   Your children

   Your extended family

   Friends

   Co-workers

   Your religious community

   God

3. Are there ways you can successfully challenge your recurring wounding thoughts?

4. Do you have the desire and skills to repair any damage to your important relationships? If not, are you willing to seek help?

5. What regrets do you experience that cause you emotional pain?

6. Are there things you can do differently now to change your tomorrows and reduce your regrets and emotional pain?

Chapter 30

Thoughts and Emotions That Heal

Experiencing the same event with a different perspective can make the difference between thoughts that wound and thoughts that heal. For example, when I initially went to my urologist for a simple prescription refill, I expected it to be the easiest doctor's appointment in my life. It didn't turn out that way. During that exam, he found a lump that he said could be cancer. For many months, I thought of that appointment as the worst doctor's visit in my lifetime.

Six months later I looked back on that exam and felt gratitude toward the doctor who performed a digital exam when it wasn't medically necessary. I now consider that appointment the best of my life. As a result, my prostate cancer was diagnosed early, while it was contained in my prostate. I'm now cured of cancer, in part because that doctor insisted on a prostate exam when all I wanted and needed was a prescription refill. The worst appointment of my life was transformed into the best because of a change in my perspective. Nothing about the exam changed—it was my change in perspective that made all the difference.

I'll provide another personal example. In this instance, one of my unhealthy fears was transformed into courage. Unhealthy fear causes emotional pain, avoidance, and paralysis. Healthy fear gives birth to an important character trait called courage. Courage is not the absence of fear but the willingness to move forward and do what's needed in the presence of fear. My willingness to learn and then perform penile injections in spite of my fear was an act of courage.

God understands we are people who often give in to our fears. I suspect that's the reason the expressions "fear not" or "do not fear" appear frequently in the Bible. Stop and think about the areas of your life that are controlled by fear. Write them down, and get a vision of what you would do in each circumstance if you were certain you could defeat fear by acting courageously. If you cannot act courageously on your own, get help from your team so you can act with courage and defeat your fears. Find promises in the Bible that will give you strength and encouragement. Remember other times in your life when you defeated your fears and acted with courage.

The diagnosis of prostate cancer will change many of your relationships. Whether that change is for the better or worse is not dependent upon your circumstances, diagnosis, or prognosis. It depends upon the life skills you and your partner possess and your personal and relational history with regard to coping with disruptive events. For example, if you or your partner have a history of using anger to resolve conflicts or one of you shuts down and gets silent and withdrawn, you can expect those behaviors to appear as you cope with the stress of dealing with prostate cancer.

There are stressful points in the journey toward surgery. How you cope with each of these stress points is important. They set the stage and framework for how you will react and cope with the next phase.

My wife worked on an oncology unit as an RN, and I had worked as a medical social worker. We've seen many people die from cancer. The images we both had were frightening. While our anxiety and fear were off the charts, we were not paralyzed by these emotions. We immediately began to educate ourselves about the disease and treatment options. We also prayed. By doing both, we no longer felt helpless. We moved from being passive to being proactive.

Here were some of our healthy core beliefs as we began our journey:

- ♦ God will use our experience with prostate cancer for our good and the good of others.

- ♦ God will comfort us.

- ♦ My wife and I will get through this.

- ♦ There is much I will learn about God, love, and life as this journey unfolds.

- ♦ I have friends I can depend on.

- ♦ If I need help, I'll seek it out.

- ♦ Laughter is good for our souls. I'll maintain a humorous perspective whenever possible.

- ♦ The reminder of my mortality contains important and valuable life lessons.

- ♦ Prayers matter and make a difference—not necessarily in receiving a positive outcome but in strengthening our faith and providing us with peace.

- ♦ Talking to other people further along this road will be extremely valuable.

- ♦ It's important to discover ways to experience gratitude. That might sound like a bad joke. Why should you be grateful when you have prostate cancer? The reason is simple: it's healthy to do so.

Here's a list of some things I was grateful for:

- ✓ That my cancer was detected early.

- ✓ That I live in an era and in a country where so many different treatment options are available.

- ✓ For highly skilled surgeons.

✓ For the opportunity to choose a great hospital.

✓ For pain medications.

✓ To have so many different choices of pads and diapers to choose from.

✓ For ED medications.

✓ For Kegels, which could help restore urinary control.

✓ For a very supportive wife.

✓ For supportive friends and family.

✓ For supportive people in online prostate cancer groups.

✓ For the good books and authors who wrote about prostate cancer.

✓ For a great pathology report.

✓ For faith that sustained and comforted me.

✓ To God, who works all things together for my good.

Maintaining thoughts that heal is a difficult task. There were phases in this journey when I became overwhelmed with negativity and thoughts that wound. This could happen to you as well. There will be times you'll need people on your team to hold you because the burden is too heavy. It's healthy to admit you are overwhelmed and need the support of others and from God.

Some promises from the Bible were very helpful to me, including:

"For God has not given us a spirit of fear, but of power and of love and of a sound mind" (2 Timothy 1:7).

"For I know the thoughts that I think toward you, says the LORD, thoughts of peace and not of evil, to give you a future and a hope. Then you will call upon me and go and pray to me, and I will listen to you. And you will seek me and find me, when you search for me with all your heart" (Jeremiah 29:11–13).

"Let us therefore come boldly to the throne of grace, that we may obtain mercy and find grace to help in time of need" (Hebrews 4:16).

"God is our refuge and strength, a very present help in trouble. Therefore we will not fear, even though the earth be removed, and though the mountains be carried into the midst of the sea; though its waters roar and be troubled, Though the mountains shake with its swelling" (Psalm 46:1–3).

Questions to Consider

1. How have you as a couple coped with other crises in your life?

2. When have you been successful helping one another in the past?

3. Can you use those skills and lessons and apply them to this situation? If so, how, and if not, why not?

4. Do you have other sources of support, such as friends, family, your faith, your religious community, and a prostate cancer support group (either online or in person)?

5. How can you bring those sources of support into your current situation?

6. How can your faith strengthen you during this time?

Chapter 31

The Expectation Gap

I found an unexpected and unpleasant surprise as I reentered the world postprostate surgery. I call this phenomenon the "expectation gap." The expectation gap develops because a rapid healing with robotic surgery takes place. Barring any complications, from all outward appearances, it will look as though you've fully recovered within a month. If you are as fortunate as I was, you'll be told no further treatment because the cancer was confined to your prostate.

Within that time frame my friends and family made two highly inaccurate assumptions. Assumption one: I was fully recovered from surgery. Assumption two: My life returned to normal. Nothing could have been further from the truth. My life had not returned to anything that resembled normal.

I thought surgery damaged the quality of my life beyond repair. There was no doubt in my mind choosing surgery was the worst decision I'd made in my lifetime. There were times I thought I'd have been better off not treating prostate cancer, living my life to the fullest, and allowing the disease to take it's course, even if that meant dying of prostate cancer. I've known some men who received the fantastic news surgery cured them of cancer, yet they were so discouraged with the quality of their life, they thought about suicide.

For every man facing these struggles, there is a wide gap between how your friends and family feel, how they expect you to feel, and how you are actually feeling. My friends and family were relieved, grateful and delighted I healed from surgery and was cured from cancer. They assumed I felt the same way. Nothing could be further from the truth. I was in the process of falling off an emotional cliff. I hated every waking moment of my life. I felt alone and isolated. Those two feelings are highly dangerous when they are paired with thoughts of suicide. If you have thoughts about killing yourself, do not keep these thoughts a secret. Please seek out professional help because you are seriously depressed.

My first attempt to bridge the expectation gap was a dismal failure. I realized this after I received an angry e-mail from a friend asking me why I still thought I needed emotional support when I'd healed from surgery and my battle with cancer was over. I never bothered to answer that e-mail. I came to the conclusion that e-mail characterized the way healthy people viewed my situation. I gave up on the idea my healthy friends or family could possibly understand the emotional impact of living life without a prostate.

I became so depressed I didn't want to see a happy face, have someone tell me how good I looked, or hear someone tell me how glad they were that I was cured of cancer. I wanted my friends and family to be happy for me, but I was incapable of sharing their joy. I didn't want to bring their mood down, or explain how and why I felt so miserable after I received the news I was cured of cancer. I came to the conclusion there was no way to bridge this expectation gap. Therefore, I limited my contact with people to the men I'd met on-line who were coping with similar issues.

I remain uncertain whether my decision to maintain the

expectation gap was the right thing to do. If you experience this expectation gap post-surgery, you will feel temporarily isolated from your friends and family. You may find this gap especially painful in the groups you belong to, such as your religious community or place of employment.

I have a suggestion, if you'd like to bridge the expectation gap. When someone approaches you with a congratulatory remark such as, "Isn't it wonderful to be cured of cancer?," you can agree that it is wonderful and add that your post-surgery life is more difficult than you expected. If that person follows up with a question or shows some interest, you can decide whether to share a difficulty you are facing. I'm convinced it is vitally important you find people and places where you can honestly share your pre-surgical and post-surgical fears, concerns, and issues.

Looking back, there were a variety of reasons I shut Brenda out of my life. One reason was Brenda was a healthy person who was glad I was alive, at a time I was wishing I hadn't survived my surgery. How could I tell Brenda I'd prefer death to living together or that I was certain she'd be better off without me. I thought it best to keep these awful thoughts to myself. As a result of my keeping secrets, Brenda and I lost many opportunities to offer each other our love, guidance, wisdom and support. Based on my experiences with self-imposed isolation, I offer this advice; be willing to share whatever is in your heart. Stay close to your partner especially through the times you are tempted to push away. It's a difficult journey and both you and your partner need all the love and support you can offer to one another.

Questions to Consider

1. Do you have people in your life you'd prefer remain unaware of your struggles post-surgery?

2. How is the expectation gap affecting your relationship with them?

3. How will you decide whether or not to bridge the expectation gap?

4. Who do you feel safe enough with, to bridge the expectation gap? (If the answer is no one, please visit our website: whereisyourprostate.com)

Chapter 32

Returning to Work

You may feel extremely self-conscious at work. From outward appearances, your co-workers will think you've healed completely. Therefore, the expectation gap may be present at your place of employment. Your co-workers and management have no idea about the emotional trauma you face living in diapers and/or coping with erectile dysfunction and marital stress. You may be returning to work at a time when you are severely depressed and/or sleeping poorly.

From my discussions with men regarding the issue of returning to work, I think the most frequent mistake men make is to return too soon. I've known men who went back to work two weeks after surgery. Many of those men expressed regret they returned so quickly.

I think there are a number of reasons for wanting to return as soon as possible. The first is related to the cost of staying home and not collecting a paycheck. The second has to do with hoping work will be an escape from all the painful emotions swirling around in your head. The third is a desire to get some things back into your life that is familiar. Lastly, work provides men with an area of your life you can control.

Going back to work when you are dealing with urinary incontinence is extremely stressful. You may not feel ready to return for an extended period if you are coping with severe incontinence. Two weeks after surgery, I was still wetting through my pants multiple times a day. There was no way I was ready or willing to go back to work.

If you dealing with severe urinary incontinence or struggling emotionally in a way that would affect your job performance, you can ask your urologist to delay clearing you for work. Many states offer some type of disability program. As long as you are not medically cleared, you may be eligible to receive disability benefits, which can reduce the financial pressures.

If you do return to work, you will be told not to perform tasks that involve heavy lifting for four to six weeks. If your job requires heavy lifting, notify your surgeon. If your employer does not have light-duty work available for you, it will be necessary for you to take a minimum of four weeks off. Your surgeon will tell you when you can safely lift heavy items. Trust his or her judgment in this matter.

I began working at home the day after I returned from the hospital. I found this task easy because it involved sitting in a chair and using my computer. I am self-employed. I own two sandwich shops. I've been through many surgeries, and I've made sure my shops can get along fine without me. Doing bookwork at home while sitting on a reclining chair and talking on the phone was not difficult to do shortly after surgery. I expected I'd be back at my restaurants within a month. However, my urinary incontinence was so severe that I stayed home for three months.

My experience was unusual. Most men can return within one month. This means the majority of those men will need to wear a pad or a diaper. They'll also need access to a bathroom in order to change every few hours. I'd suggest bringing at least one change of clothing in case you leak through and wet your pants.

If you or management notice your performance has fallen below company standards, it's important to explain to management that while it appears you are fully recovered, there are many issues you are facing that may be affecting your job performance. Taking additional time off, or temporarily changing job responsibilities may become necessary.

If you can afford it, I think it's better to err on the side of caution. My advice is to resist the temptation to return to work as early as possible. Stay home until you experience some relief and healing from the physical and emotional trauma that occur after prostate surgery.

Questions to Consider/ Things to do

1. If your state has a disability program, have you applied for this benefit?

2. If your job involves heaving lifting, you need to make arrangements for light duty until your surgeon says it is safe for you to lift heavy items.

3. Do you feel pressure to return to work? If so, Why?

4. Do you plan to bridge the expectation gap with anyone? If so, why so? If not, why not?

5. If you are experiencing severe sleep disruption make sure you are not involved in long distance driving or operating dangerous equipment and ask your surgeon for medical clearance before you resume these tasks.

Chapter 33

Characteristics of Good Comfort

But I would strengthen you with my mouth, and the comfort of my lips would relieve your grief.—Job 16:5

There are people in your day-to-day life, perhaps co-workers, who possess the wisdom, skills, and ability to provide you with good comfort. These are people you want on your team.

When you've received good comfort, you experience one or more of the following:

♦ **Offers understanding.** Good comfort is not about finding just the right words to say in the attempt to make the person suffering or the comforter feel better. It's a willingness to listen without interrupting. There's a freedom to delve as deeply into your experiences as you need to go. With understanding words and/or nonverbal behavior, you know the person beside you is with you on your journey.

♦ **Offers compassion.** There is a temptation to distance ourselves when someone is suffering. Compassion is the willingness to suffer along with someone in pain or need. Compassion may but doesn't necessarily move us to do something to help or relieve suffering.

♦ **Instills hope.** To instill hope means someone can look to the future and imagine and experience time beyond his or her current suffering. He or she can experience some relief or perspective and look optimistically at a better future.

♦ **Offers empathy.** Involves a willingness to walk in someone's shoes for a while. It involves a willingness to hear about and understand what another person is feeling.

♦ **Moves you toward rather than away from other people.** When someone takes the time to be with you in meaningful ways, your desire for social contact increases.

♦ **Brings you closer to God.** When you have the faith to believe God loves you regardless of the outcome or success with treatment, dark times can draw you closer to God than good times ever will.

♦ **Lightens the load.** This will happen when some people offer to help you in any meaningful way. Preparing a meal or giving any form of practical assistance can offer relief.

♦ **Stays in touch.** Few if any people who began this journey with you will stay in touch throughout the whole ordeal. Expect that and appreciate the imperfect ways people stay connected.

♦ **Never judges but may confront.** No one likes to be judged and found guilty in the eyes of another person. Judgment is frequently a negative evaluation about your character based on a behavior. For example, after surgery, you begin to withdraw from your wife. A judgmental remark would be, "Why are you acting so selfishly by only thinking about yourself?" Calling your husband selfish is judgmental. The same behavior of withdrawal can be confronted without being judgmental. For example, a wife could share that she misses her husband's company. She expresses her need for him to be there for her and how much she misses his presence, strength, and love.

There's another important source of comfort, which was the most important source of comfort I received. I'm speaking of the comfort Brenda and I received from God. It is easy to miss God's comfort when we are overwhelmed with fear and anxiety. Sometimes we only see it looking back, but we may miss it in the moment. Additionally, it's easy to become angry or disappointed with the comfort God offers to us. This happens when we expect God to use His power to prevent a tragedy or illness from happening.

Here are some of the places you will find comfort from God:

- ◆ **From God's Word.** There are many promises and words of comfort found in the Old and New Testaments.

- ◆ **From God's people.** God will bring special people into your life. If you have no belief in God, you will say, "I was lucky to have met them." If you have faith, you will thank God for those people.

- ◆ **From prayer.** It would take an entire book to discuss the value of prayer. Don't neglect your relationship with God during this crisis. Prayer invites God into your circumstances.

- ◆ **From God's promises.** It's not God's intention to waste a single moment of your suffering. Understanding His promises to you in your suffering doesn't take away the pain but gives meaning to it. Suffering is a vivid reminder that our times in this world and in our bodies are both temporary.

- ◆ **From God's presence.** I believe the covenant God

made with both Jews and Christians means God is present and shares in our suffering in ways that are beyond our understanding. He is not a God who watches our suffering from a distance.

♦ **From God's purpose.** Suffering without meaning leads to despair. Suffering with meaning invites growth and purpose into your life. Not everyone will grow as a result of suffering.

♦ **From God's provision.** When God calls you to go through anything, He provides what's necessary. If the manna God gave the Jewish people in the wilderness is a picture of His provision—and I think it is—this means we will receive enough for twenty-four hours, not for twenty-one or twenty-six. We receive our provisions for each new day. God is faithful and does not skip a day. It's up to us to take the time to gather these provisions.

♦ **From the Holy Spirit.** A person is sealed with the Holy Spirit when he or she accepts Jesus as his or her Savior. The Holy Spirit guides, teaches, convicts, enables, and provides spiritual fruit, such as love, joy, peace, patience, kindness, goodness, faithfulness, and self-control.

♦ **From hymns and praise songs.** Brenda and I immediately found comfort from hymns and praise songs. I appreciated songs such as "It Is Well with My Soul," "Blessed Be Your Name," "Jesus Messiah," "Hold on, Help Is on the Way," "The Blessing," and a host of others. There were many days I spent hours a day listening to those songs and singing along. Here are some that meant the most to me:

Michael Smith, "Help Is on the Way"[3]

---

3 http://www.youtube.com/watch?v=OcjjT-8Zc3U.

Laura Story, "Blessings"[4]

Newsboys, "Blessed Be Your Name"[5]

♦ **From the prayers of other people**. Brenda and I felt uplifted and encouraged by the people we knew who were praying for us.

♦ **From answered prayers**. There were decisions we had to make that we took to prayer. We believe we received guidance when we did this. Throughout my journey with prostate cancer, my faith in the Lord made a huge difference in my life. He can and will do this in yours if you ask Him.

Questions to Consider

1. Can you find comfort in your faith? If so, how so?

2. If not, why not?

3. Is prayer a source of comfort to you? If so, how so? If not, Why not?

4. Is the word of God a source of comfort to you? If so, share this with your partner.

5. If not, is that something that interests you at this time?

6. Are there any types of music, which provides comfort to you?

7. If you have no faith in God, are your experiences with cancer calling you toward or pushing you away from seeking God?

---

4 http://www.youtube.com/watch?v=1CSVqHcdhXQ.

5 http://www.youtube.com/watch?v=DLycgKxIgc0.

Chapter 34

Characteristics of Miserable Comfort

I have heard many such things; miserable comforters are you all! Shall words of wind have an end?—Job 16:2–3

Unfortunately, many people lack the skills to provide comfort. This isn't a new problem; it's been going on throughout history. More than two thousand years ago, a man named Job suffered a series of tragic events. His friends came to comfort him. After experiencing their comfort, he told them the truth: they were "miserable comforters." I wouldn't advise you to repeat that phrase to anyone, but the odds are the words miserable comforter will come to your mind more than once.

Some of your friends and family mean well, but they lack comforting skills. Even with their best efforts, the comfort they provide will be miserable.

Here are some characteristics of miserable comfort:

❖ **Judges you.** In one way or another, your comforter will blame you for the trouble and pain you are going through. "If you'd have eaten more fish, maybe you wouldn't have prostate cancer."

❖ **Misunderstands you.** "Why are you afraid of prostate cancer? You are going to a top treatment center."

❖ **Wrongly directs your attention.** "My dad died from prostate cancer."

❖ **Frustrates and/or exasperates you.** "You don't need surgery; just drink loads of pomegranate juice."

❖ **Leaves you feeling misunderstood.** "What's the big deal about having your prostate removed?"

❖ **Separates or disconnects you from God and/or other people.** "Why are you angry with God? That's a sin."

❖ **Increases your pain or suffering.** "Stop whining like a baby. You'll be fine."

❖ **Shifts attention away from the sufferer to the comforter.** "When I had prostate surgery, they didn't know about sparing nerve bundles. You're lucky."

❖ **Leaves you feeling you are better off suffering alone and/or angry with your comforter.** "This is a blessing in disguise; God will work this out for your good." A comment such as this is theologically correct but demonstrates no sense of empathy.

❖ **Offers comfort clichés.** You've been hit with a comfort cliché when someone offers a sentence or two that comforts him or her, not you. Typically the person who gives the comfort cliché walks away as quickly as possible, too afraid to find out how you're really doing. He or she might say, "I'll pray for you" but never asks you what you need prayer for. Another example is someone who offers some positive way to look at things. For example, "Forget about the things that bother you; look at the bright side of life." Remember that the goal of the person offering the comfort cliché is to avoid hearing how you are really doing, so don't make the mistake of attempting to share intimate parts of your life with a person who offers you a comfort cliché. Thank him or her for the good wishes and move on.

There is an opportunity—and I can't say this enough times—for you to seek out new team members further along the journey of prostate cancer. If you seek these people out, you will be pleasantly surprised to experience the way in which strangers are able to provide you with information, help, and support and will comfort you in ways you find invaluable.

Questions to Consider

1. Can you predict in advance who will be a miserable comforter? How will this affect your expectations of them?

2. How will you deal with those who offer miserable comfort?

3. Discuss the times when both of you have provided miserable comfort to each other?

4. Discuss what you have learned from those experiences?

5. Are there things you need to change in order to stop providing miserable comfort to each other?

Chapter 35

Lessons Learned about Comfort

I learned some important lessons from my experiences receiving good, bad, and no comfort. There were some people in my life who had a history of providing good and meaningful comfort for those things I was willing to share. There was one important exception to this. When I tried to share post-surgical issues with healthy men and women, it didn't go well. They had no frame of reference to relate to the experiences and issues I was coping with. Therefore, I limited my sharing of post-surgical issues to men who had prostate cancer. They were able to empathize with my struggles.

Here are some lessons I learned:

♦ Don't expect people to be there for you if there wasn't a history of them being there in the past. The fact you could be facing a life-threatening illness does not mean people will rally to help you in any way. This is true even when those people share your last name. There are some people in my family I didn't even tell about my having cancer because we've been estranged for decades.

♦ Even people close to you will at times let you

down. Don't take it personally or allow a single disappointment to ruin or end those relationships.

♦ When I became severely depressed, I withdrew from everyone, including my wife. At that point, I was unable to receive or provide good comfort to my wife. My decision to isolate myself and withdraw from everyone prolonged my suffering.

♦ Spend time with people you can have fun and/ or laugh with. Sometimes I needed a break from thinking about cancer or dealing with the aftermath of surgery.

♦ Some of the best comfort will come from those further along in the journey. Make sure you find ways to meet men and couples who've been through this together.

♦ I can't begin to explain how much the prayers of others aided Brenda and me through this journey. Find people who will pray for you.

♦ God is a God of good comfort. Sometimes you can miss it. Sometimes you may not experience it in a way you understand or hope for, but believe it's there and available to you and for you.

♦ God's comfort doesn't necessarily mean your suffering will end. It means you can and will suffer in a different way.

♦ Remember to pray. The Bible teaches us that sometimes we miss out on God's blessings because we haven't asked for them in prayer. Don't expect God to provide you with a happily-ever-after ending on this side of eternity.

♦ In order to receive comfort, you have to take risks and share what's going on. Test the waters, and go slowly. If you receive bad comfort, move on. Eventually you'll find people with the time, skills, willingness, and ability to provide good comfort.

♦ Allow your experiences to mold you into a good comforter. Also know that good comforters sometimes miss the mark. Don't expect anyone, including yourself, to have the capacity to provide good comfort one hundred percent of the time.

♦ Prepare yourself for some unpleasant surprises. You will experience some unexpected hurts and disappointments from friends or family. When someone demonstrates to you by word or deed that he or she is unable to provide good comfort, believe that person! If you can, enjoy other aspects of that relationship.

♦ Prepare yourself for pleasant surprises. When you least expect it, someone will bless you.

♦ Good comfort, acts of kindness, and meaningful prayer will come from people and other places you could not have predicted or expected.

An example of this came from my meeting a man online through a prostate cancer support group. We discovered we both lived in California but hundreds of miles apart. It turned out both of us chose UCSF for our surgery. We also discovered we had the same surgeon. Later we found we had appointments at UCSF on the same day within thirty minutes of each other. We decided to meet in the waiting room at UCSF. When we met, we talked as if we'd known each other for years. Since that day, he and I and our wives have stayed in touch, supporting and praying for each other. All of us realized the infinitesimal odds of this happening. We all agreed it was the Lord who had brought us together.

In order for these surprises to occur, you can't be sitting home alone waiting for them to happen. If I had not reached out to an online prostate cancer support group, we would not have met this couple.

Another example was a renewal of an old friendship

dating back more than thirty years. We hadn't been in touch for decades. We reconnected via Facebook. It's been an amazing blessing for this friendship to be renewed.

It is important for you and your partner to take the time and be purposeful in developing sources for good comfort. You will miss out on receiving support and good comfort if you act passively and assume people will rally around you once they hear you have cancer. Good comfort will enable you to work through the difficult issues you must cope with before and after surgery.

Questions/Thoughts to Consider

1. Who in your life has provided you with good comfort?

2. What qualities and skills do those people possess?

3. Discuss your history of providing good comfort to one another.

4. Identify the skills you both possess to successfully provide good comfort to each other?

5. Identify the skills you need to learn in order to provide good comfort to each other?

6. Develop a plan to receive good comfort.

7. What lessons are you learning about giving and receiving good comfort?

Chapter 36

Time to Sing a New Song

At eighteen months post-surgery, I didn't realize how stressed our relational life was until I showed my wife a post from a cancer support forum. This woman shared her distress that her husband was pulling away from her emotionally after his surgery. I asked Brenda how our life experiences could help her. I had no idea at the time I'd asked a loaded question. My wife didn't think we could help at all because we were going through the same crisis.

Like most men, I was oblivious to this news, and we had a two-day-long fight over this issue. During that time, I learned how much emotional pain Brenda continued to experience because she felt I was still emotionally and physically withdrawn.

I thought I was doing much better than Brenda felt I was. However, after hearing Brenda's perspective on our relationship, I realized I had not come as far as I thought I had. We needed to intentionally work on our marriage every day.

We took a vacation together, which added a great deal of fun, new experiences, and time for romance. We had a fantastic time together. We needed that downtime away from the responsibility and pressures of everyday life. Our vacation brought us closer together.

Songs often remind us of important emotional or relational periods in our lives. After this argument, I realized a verse from the song "Yesterday," sung by Paul McCartney, became my post-surgical theme song. Those lyrics were, "Suddenly, I'm not half the man I used to be." As "half a man," I truly believed my wife would be better off without me. I came to the realization I didn't feel I deserved Brenda's love or dedication. I genuinely thought she would be better off with someone else, a man who was whole.

For eighteen consecutive months I'd failed my wife physically and relationally. I was feeling so bad about myself, that if our marriage were a contract, I would have advised her to leave me. Fortunately and thankfully, our marriage is not a contractual agreement. In the book of Genesis, God created the institution of marriage to be a lifelong covenant. When we promised each other to stay together till "death do us part," that promise was part of the covenant we made with each other. While I agreed with Brenda that I had failed to love her the way she deserved, I also believed with all my heart that with God's help, Brenda and I have yet to live the best years of our marriage.

This could not and would not happen if I continued to base my identity and manhood on my sexuality and performance in the bedroom. If I continued on this path, it was possible the verse from "Yesterday" would become my theme song forever.

In order to sing a new song, I did not want to wait until my circumstances changed. I knew it was time to renew my mind and see things from a different perspective. I turned to the Bible and focused on verses that reminded me who I was in Christ. Here were a few verses that spoke to me:

"You are the salt of the earth" (Matthew 5:13).

"You are the light of the world" (Matthew 5:14).

"But you are a chosen generation, a royal priesthood, a

holy nation, His own special people, that you may proclaim the praises of Him who called you out of darkness into His marvelous light" (1 Peter 2:9).

"No longer do I call you servants, for a servant does not know what his master is doing; but I have called you friends" (John 15:15).

"Therefore, if anyone is in Christ, he is a new creation; old things have passed away; behold, all things have become new" (2 Corinthians 5:17).

Keeping these and other biblical promises in mind, I was ready to sing a new song (even though it's an oldie from the sixties) by Spiral Staircase. I lined up about ten bottles of prescription and over-the-counter medication. I placed them on the counter in our bathroom. Then I called Brenda into the room. I used my phone to access YouTube. com. As the song played, I used the different bottles of medication to make different sounds to the beat of the song. I wanted to use humor to make an important point. The bottles of medication were visual reminders of all the physical changes and challenges the years have brought to me and to us. Yet through it all, laughter and love could and would continue to flourish.

These are the lyrics to the song I chose as my new theme song: "Oh, I love you more today than yesterday. But not as much as tomorrow!"[6]

Questions/Thoughts to Consider

1. Choose a song that best describes how you feel following surgery. Is that the song you want to

---

6 "I Love You More Today" by Spiral Staircase: http://www.youtube.com/watch?v=ec1vK-LEJs8&feature=results_video&playnext=1&list=PLBC82A6EA4CFF0591.

be your theme song in the months and years to come?

2. Is there another song you'd prefer as a theme song? What needs to happen for you to make it your new song?

Chapter 37

Forever Healed

The natural world frequently teaches us a truth about the spiritual world. I believe this applies to prostate cancer. Before your prostate cancer was diagnosed, it is likely cancer cells were growing in your prostate for a long time without your knowledge. In other words, for many years you had a potentially life-threatening disease, but you spent those years unaware and mistakenly believing you were in good health.

In the very same way, there are many people without an understanding of the consequences of living their lives separated from God due to sin. They are unaware of the danger they face in that condition. Like prostate cancer, there may be no obvious symptoms. From the outside looking in, many people without a relationship with God live successful lives. They enjoy long-term marriages. They raise wonderful children. They might have highly successful careers, make a lot of money, and enjoy many material things. They can be rich, famous, and influential in our world. Success often drives us away from God.

From the opposite direction, there are many people who've made a mess of their lives. Some come from broken families and repeat destructive lifestyles they'd hoped to escape. Others had terrible things happen to them, which resulted in their making poor life choices. Some folks feel so awful about themselves they can't conceive of a heavenly Father who loves them. This becomes challenging if your earthly father was abusive or abandoned the family. Success, tragedy, and a host of other life experiences move us away from a relationship with God.

When I first received the diagnosis of prostate cancer, one of the first questions that popped into my mind was whether cancer would kill me. The concept of dying was not mysterious to me. The Bible tells us exactly what happens the moment we die: "For we walk by faith, not by sight. We are confident, yes, well pleased rather to be absent from the body and to be present with the Lord" (2 Corinthians 5:7–8).

The truth was I didn't feel pleased with the idea of being absent from my body. I wasn't ready to die. I've always dreamed of the day when I would walk my daughter down the aisle. I'm a tad over protective when it comes to my daughter. I warned her I was capable of handcuffing us together as we walked down the aisle. After a great deal of fussing and crying, I hoped I would be willing to uncuff us, so the wedding could proceed. I wanted to live long enough to see all four of our children married. I wanted the opportunity to become a grandparent. I wanted to live long enough to enjoy many years of retirement with my wife. The possibility I'd miss some or all of these events caused me great sorrow and a lot of tears.

Eventually, I reached a place of peace, trusting God's timing when I'd receive the call to be absent from my body and present with the Lord. With that peace in place, my sorrow remained. I didn't want to die of prostate cancer or miss so many important family milestones.

When I received the fantastic news that surgery cured me of prostate cancer, I experienced enormous relief. I felt as though I'd received a commutation from a death sentence. For a brief period of time, I went back to living as if death and dying were not a reality.

Prostate and colon cancer run in my family. When I turned sixty I made an appointment for a colonoscopy. During that exam two polyps were removed and sent to a lab for a biopsy.

As Brenda and I waited to receive the biopsy results from my colon polyps I was forcefully reminded a second time how quickly we can loose the blessing of good health. I came to the realization being cured from prostate cancer did not guarantee I'd live long enough to see any of those important family milestones. After facing the possibility of cancer a second time, it was burned into my consciousness healing from prostate cancer did not change the reality I remain terminal, so are you. One day, through accident, injury, illness or disease, all of us are going to die.

The Bible says: "But He was wounded for our transgressions, He was bruised for our iniquities; The chastisement for our peace was upon Him, And by His stripes we are healed." (Isaiah 53:5) I've personally experienced this healing. It's a far greater healing than prostate surgery could ever provide. It's a healing that lasts throughout eternity. I don't know how many hours that you will spend investigating the various treatment options before you'll come to a decision about how to treat your prostate cancer.

Choosing your treatment option could be one of the most difficult decisions you'll make in your lifetime. Take the necessary time, and make your decision wisely. Whether you are dealing with a curable or a life-threatening cancer may be unknown to you right now. No doubt, it's a time when you and your family are coping with an enormous amount of stress.

Therefore, what I'm about to say may be hard for you to believe. Jesus poses a far more important question than how to treat your prostate cancer. In fact, it is the most important question you'll ever answer— If you say a single word, you will experience a far greater healing than a healing from prostate cancer.

Here's the question straight from the lips of Jesus: I am the resurrection and the life. He who believes in Me, though he may die, he shall live. And whoever lives and believes in Me shall never die. Do you believe this?" (John 11:25-27)

If your answer is yes, you've defeated both prostate cancer and death! If your answer to that question was no, I'd like to respectfully ask you to spend some of your time investigating the claims and teachings of Jesus. If you don't have a Bible, I suggest you get one and start reading the first book of the New Testament, which is the book of Matthew. I've also included some additional resources listed in the bibliography to start you off.

I hope you'll visit us on our website, **whereisyourprostate. com**, I pray I will meet you face to face where:

... God will wipe away every tear from their eyes; there shall be no more death, nor sorrow, nor crying. There shall be no more pain, for the former things have passed away. Then He who sat on the throne said, "Behold, I make all things new." (Revelation 21:4–5).

God has the last word on our pain, suffering, illness, disease, and death—and it is good!

Chapter 38

Afterthoughts

I've taken you on my journey with prostate cancer and surgery. I've shared how this disease affected my emotional, psychological, relational, sexual, and spiritual life. If this were not a God-ordained ministry, I would never have shared many of the experiences I've written about with anyone other than my wife. Both of us believe we were called to share our private and intimate experiences in order to assist others facing similar issues find ways to talk about their struggles following prostate surgery.

I was clueless and unprepared regarding ways surgery would affect me. As a result, I suffered, my wife suffered, and our marriage suffered. There are enough studies out there that show how depressed men become after prostate surgery, yet there is little or no preparation or discussion about post-surgical depression. Men who are about to make a decision that will permanently alter the quality of their lives should be exposed to more than glitzy ads, ridiculous claims, and meaningless statistics. I thought I'd breeze through surgery and heal quickly. When my expectations and timetable were proved wrong, my profound disappointment fueled my emotional and relational suffering.

After surgery, I wondered when I'd think of myself as healed from prostate cancer. Early on, I thought healing from prostate cancer meant months would go by without my experiencing a passing thought about prostate cancer.

This never happened. While I don't worry about the return of prostate cancer, I think of myself as a prostate cancer survivor every day. It's become part of my identity. Prostate cancer is not something I need to forget about in order to think I have finally healed.

I didn't expect I'd become a man on a mission. I encourage men to have their yearly prostate exams and PSA tests. I never wanted to be a blogger, yet now I blog about prostate cancer at: http://whereisyourprostate. blogspot.com/. It wasn't in my life plan to write a book about prostate cancer, yet here it is. Most men with prostate cancer will find themselves called to be a resource in their circle of friends and acquaintances. Don't be surprised if you are asked to contact a friend of a friend who was just diagnosed.

How prostate cancer or any other disruptive moment affects your life and your relationships is up to you. I've known men who decided to live selfishly after they were diagnosed. It didn't matter whether their marriages stayed together or failed. When their marriages did fail, these men were relieved or unconcerned.

I've heard from men and/or their wives who remain angry or bitter years after surgery. They still struggle with issues they thought would resolve in a few short months. From the other direction, I've known couples who've managed to grow stronger in the face of permanent loss of urinary control and/or erectile dysfunction.

The good news is that the fate and future of your most important relationships are not necessarily dependent on a positive surgical outcome or being cured of cancer. Emotional connections, intimacy, and the capacity to enjoy relationships with people and with God are all possible in every circumstance.

Whether you become bitter or better is based upon

a series of choices you make. I believe the best way to prepare yourself for your post-surgical life is to be prepared, ready, willing, and able to face the worst possible outcome while holding out hope for a better outcome. Nineteen months after my surgery, I can say I don't want my prostate back, and I made the right choice to treat my prostate cancer. I believe this even though on occasion, I'll leak urine and my response to ED medication is still hit and miss. In other words, I'm still glad I chose surgery even though I continue to experience post-surgical issues.

If you are interested in hearing from other men who've had surgery, I invite you to check out and/or participate in a survey about prostate surgery at http://www.whereisyourprostate.com/Forums.html and to join a forum as well. Whatever way you choose to treat your prostate cancer, I pray years down the road, you'll believe you made the right decision.

Part II:
Brenda's Chapters

Chapter 39

Praying for the Blessing

While waiting for our daughter, Kate, to get out of her college class, I often turned on the Christian radio station. On this particular day, a week prior to Rick's upcoming surgery, I had asked God to provide comfort and to prevent a bad situation from occurring in our family. Rick had just been diagnosed with prostate cancer. Almost two months of waiting had passed for his surgery date. Much soul searching and worry had already passed. I felt terror the day the doctor called to tell Rick he had cancer. I broke down in tears. Flooded with emotion, I attempted to tell our family. While still sore and overwhelmed, I was looking for gifts from God.

Then I heard a song playing in the background, and my heart was immediately touched. Laura Story's song "The Blessing" spoke volumes to me. She and her husband were newlyweds, and her husband had been diagnosed two years earlier with a brain tumor with complications of encephalitis. As she attempted to sort out and understand what had just happened, she reflected they had prayed for healing but didn't get the answer they wanted. She began questioning and processing the reasons God had not answered her prayers the way she'd requested.[7]

I love this song because it doesn't try to sugarcoat or dismiss the hardness of her situation. It doesn't throw out the platitudes we often hear from our fellow believers that attempt to lessen the angst of the messenger while leaving the sufferer suffering more. Laura's thoughts show genuine opinion and feelings, both of which God could handle even when fellow believers or family may not. Yet it brought me fear. Would this happen to Rick and me? We too had not gotten the answer we wanted when we prayed—Rick was still diagnosed with cancer. I so didn't want this to happen. Like Laura, I searched for answers. I wondered if our suffering was a blessing in disguise. [7]

Rick and I were now in the middle of a crisis. I found myself with a great need of God's mighty hand to ease our suffering and heal Rick. We prayed, and we asked for prayer. To all of you who prayed for us, I thank you once again! Prayer is significant to me. During the initial moments of our crisis, prayer made a difference. Prayer means different things to each of us. For some it is profound, for others it's a ritual, and for others still it doesn't have anything to do with them. I invite you in your journey to consider whether prayer has any significance for you. I was feeling so unsafe and threatened that I slipped into hyper-vigilance, a familiar place. I needed so much courage, reminders I was not alone, strength, faith, and comfort. Some are able to slip into denial, but that has never been my way. I needed help. I prayed. Through prayer God reminded me, as I felt the intensity of cancer, *I am here.*

My favorite verse of late helps me remember during the stresses: "And He said, 'My presence will go with you, and I will give you rest'" (Exodus 33:14).

---

7 http://www.youtube.com/results?search_query=the+blessing+la ura+story+behind+the+song&oq=the+blessing+laura+story+behin d+the+song&gs_l=youtube.3 ... 4088.9732.0.9864.16.15.0.0.0.0.18 2.1475.8j6.14.0 ... 0.0 ... 1ac.DS6J-gVJRWk.

Through prayer, God also reminds me to tell Him what is important to me. He tells us, "So I say to you, ask, and it will be given to you; seek, and you will find; knock, and it will be opened to you. For everyone who asks receives" (Luke 11:9–10).

"The LORD will guide you continually, and satisfy your soul in drought, and strengthen your bones; you shall be like a watered garden, and like a spring of water, whose waters do not fail" (Isaiah 58:11).

Psalm 103:4–5 reminds us that it is God "Who redeems your life from destruction, who crowns you with lovingkindness and tender mercies, who satisfies your mouth with good things, so that your youth is renewed like the eagle's."

From these verses, I'm reminded God has promised to satisfy my needs and fill me with love and mercy. At a time when I realize I have come to the end of myself and in this situation am totally helpless, I need God. Prayer allows me to be safe and allows my voice to be heard. I find prayer to be significant because it helps me see who I am trusting.

God promises, "He shall regard the prayer of the destitute, and shall not despise their prayer" (Psalm 102:17).

Knowing God will respond to my prayers brings me much comfort. As I waited for Rick to heal physically and emotionally, I began praying to God using His different biblical names. As I prayed, I called on Elohim, which means mighty Creator or preserver. Other times I called on El Shaddai, which means almighty, all sufficient. Still other times I prayed to Adonai, which means Master or Lord. Praying to our God called by different names brought me more understanding of the capabilities of God. I had more confidence in Him. I trusted Him. I rested. Don't get me wrong—feelings ebbed and flowed, but I certainly felt more peace than I, a great worrier, felt under such circumstances.

If prayer makes such a difference, what hinders us from

praying for what we need? Is it a lack of trust, or the sense it doesn't matter anyway? Or is it kind of embarrassing to talk to someone we can't even see in a world that diminishes God and seeks to trust in ourselves? Mindfully listen to what inhibits you.

My own inhibitions to pray came from my experience in churches. I love fellow believers and the church, but I react negatively to the phrase, "This is not about you." I've heard this phrase in many different churches I've worshipped in. Each time I hear that phrase, I feel wounded. In order for me to pray, I'm called to share a huge, private part of myself with the Maker of the universe. I need to cry out my needs and fears pertaining to prostate cancer and all its consequences. I need to be genuine and open about my need. I don't want to be told my needs aren't important or that prayer isn't about me. God desires to provide for you and me. Let us receive from Him through prayer and with His presence in our lives.

There's another inhibition I have to deal with in speaking with fellow believers. It's wounding to my soul when I ask for prayer or comfort to be told, "Jesus is sufficient," and/or I'm advised to leave all my problems, fears, and anxieties at the cross. There is no doubt Jesus has enough grace for each and every situation. Yet these phrases shut me down. When I hear them, I know I need to keep my fears, doubts, and personal issues to myself.

I deeply desire and desperately need the freedom to speak with God honestly and share my heart. When we do this, we are open to receive a blessing and the joy that arrives with the blessing. Gary Thomas writes in *Pure Pleasure,* "We must be more sensitive and do a better job of helping fellow believers address legitimate physical needs." He explains God didn't say, "Adam, you don't need Eve, just keep looking at me." God acknowledged it was not good for man to be alone. We need God and other people as we go through life's trials.

Surely there are many hindrances to prayer. One might

be as simple as thinking, *I don't know how to pray.* You can pray what's in your heart. Express fear, anger, doubt, worry—whatever is in your heart can be spoken to God in prayer. So I prayed. I prayed for what I needed. I asked others to pray for me when I couldn't pray. I prayed for peace. I read my Bible. In Psalm 23 I see a shepherd showing me to lie down in green pastures. As I saw myself there, I could relax a while. I prayed for courage. Michael Smith's song "Help Is on the Way" says that God knows about our tears and gives us the courage to fight our fears. I prayed for strength. In a line from "Blessing," Laura Story asks for a mighty hand to ease our suffering. I prayed for trust. I prayed directly from the Bible with Psalm 56:3 "Whenever I am afraid, I will trust in you."

I prayed for comfort. Spurgeon in *Comfort for the Soul* asks, "Is your heart heavy? God knew it would be. The comfort your heart wants is treasured in the sweet assurance of our text. You are poor and needy, but he knows your need and has the exact blessing you require. Plead this promise, believe it, and you will obtain fulfillment." I prayed for healing and help. I asked God in prayer, "If you are willing, may you heal Rick." I was certain my prayer would be answered. The answer could be no, wait, or yes. I was confident whichever way this went, God was going to use this for His good. I knew God loved us regardless of Rick's outcome. I knew prayer doesn't provide us with a happily-ever-after ending on this side of heaven.

For some people, prostate cancer can bring about a crisis in faith. There is no shame in having doubts. It's important, though, to find safe people to express those doubts to so you won't get judged or condemned for expressing your doubts. Rick's illness did not cause a crisis in my faith. I never doubted God's love or goodwill toward us. I knew I had to add to my prayers that if Rick wasn't healed, we needed God's help to see the good in this experience. Whatever the future held, I knew it had a purpose.

After surgery at UCSF, it was important to get Rick

out of bed and walking around. We met a number of other men who'd had prostate surgery. Some had already received the news their cancer had spread beyond their prostates. We felt vulnerable. I wondered why some men received bad news while others received good news. I wondered what news we'd receive.

I knew those men who'd received the awful news were not loved any less by God. I also knew my prayers for healing didn't guarantee that's what would happen. I came to the conclusion that God was going to use our news, bad or good, for His glory and good was going to come out of it either way.

This verse reminds me that God was with us, whatever news we received: "Ah, Lord GOD! Behold, you have made the heavens and the earth by your great power and outstretched arm. There is nothing too hard for you" (Jeremiah 32:17–18).

Nicole Mullins in her song "My Redeemer Lives, talks about God's gentle hands that hold me when I'm broken.

James 5:15 says, "And the prayer of faith will save the sick, and the Lord will raise him up. And if he has committed sins, he will be forgiven."

One thing I have learned is that even though we've prayed to be healed, the answer may be no. God has promised good will come out of it, but it is not necessarily the good we want. His answer will be broader and wider and higher than we could ever imagine. That doesn't mean we won't be discouraged and disappointed perhaps for a while. Certainly I was discouraged, but when it is all said and done, we will look and see the good God has done for us. God makes a difference through my prayers and through the prayers of others. Some people prayed on their knees for us. One prayed in Hebrew. Sometimes I could only pray, "Help." We asked for prayers from a team who prayed when I was at a loss for words. One person prayed for peace of mind for Rick and me. Another friend stopped over with gifts, cards, and chocolates and asked God to help reassure me of His presence and to heal Rick.

These prayers from our friends touched me greatly:

> ➤ I (meaning God) do great things, and you are in good hands with me. I hear your prayer and will respond, for you are my child.

> ➤ We will keep praying, especially that the surgery will go perfectly and that Rick's recovery will be quick and uneventful. May the surgeon be encouraging after the surgery, and may peace abound in your hearts. The Lord loves Rick and all of you and promises to go before you. Love you.

> ➤ I will pray for Rick. Our God is so great, so strong, and so mighty, there's nothing He cannot do. Rest in His arms. He's our assurance every morning, our defender every night.

> ➤ I'm praying that the surgery is successful in removing all the cancer and that Rick will soon be up and about on the road to recovery, with minimal side-effects. The most important things for him are to have your companionship, understanding, encouragement, and ongoing love. May the Lord bless and encourage both you and Rick in the days and weeks ahead.

Prayers from our friends brought great strength and comfort. Amid the fears, great moments of peace occurred too. In great pain, it takes deep faith to go to our Father in need and ask for help. At times it may feel like our faith has failed. God already knows and graciously accepts us with our strong faith or our faith the size of a mustard seed. God also accepts us when we express our doubts, fears, and anger. It's a mistake to think great faith will make a painful situation go away, make our pain go away, or give us the outcome we desire. Faith carries us through our pain and through our circumstances.

My faith in God and confidence in prayer prepared me

to accept whatever Rick's pathology results were, good or bad. As Rick prepped for surgery at UCSF, we were anxious but knew God had been involved in every aspect so far and would be with us. The surgeon came out after four hours and said it was a "classic textbook surgery." The nerves had been spared, and no lymph nodes had been removed. Cautiously, he reported that it looked contained but he wouldn't know for sure until pathology came back in about ten days.

After surgery but prior to the final pathology report, we received this note with prayers: "Thanks for the update. I will continue to pray! May Rick get a good pathology report, and may his recovery astound all of you! The Lord bless you all. Love, J."

Ten days later, Rick received a call from a resident explaining that Rick was receiving a "dream pathology report that every prostate cancer patient would like to receive." The cancer was contained. He went on to say Rick's cancer was downgraded to a less-aggressive cancer, which occurs in some cases. Recurrence rates with these results are rare. We were extremely grateful to our Lord. We were amazed. We believed God had just given us an added gift of a lesser chance of cancer recurrence. Praying to God makes a difference! These prayers and the continued prayers for recovery mean a lot to us. I testify that my Redeemer lives not only for salvation but for all of life's experiences, for which He will make all things new.

Questions to Consider

1. What are your own thoughts and beliefs about the power and usefulness of prayer?

2. If you've never prayed, what has held you back?

3. What touched you the most in some of the prayers for Rick and me?

4. Are there specific prayers you'd like to pray right now?

5. Are you and your spouse able to pray together? If not, why not?

6. Would you allow this crisis to bring you both together to pray? If so, will you take the steps necessary to make that happen?

7. Are there other people you'd like to pray for you? If so, will you make a plan to contact them and ask for their prayers?

8. Would you like to ask your children to get involved in praying for you? If so, ask them to pray. You can make it a general request or ask them to pray for specifics.

9. Is there a body of like-minded believers to whom you could make a prayer request?

Chapter 40

Grief Revisited

One year after surgery, Rick and I meandered through the trails in Pacific Grove of the Monarch Butterfly Reserve. Prior to visiting, I thought we would see hundreds of free-flying butterflies. Instead, we found maybe one or two huddled close to the ground. The next day we went again, hoping, but being realistic we wouldn't see many. As we ambled down the path, we saw only Eucalyptus trees, a few pines, and scraggly bushes of some sort. Still in the shade, we saw the occasional body of a monarch that hadn't made it. But farther down, in the sun way above the trees floating high and safe, were the hundreds of gorgeous butterflies mating or at least attempting to do so. A self-prescribed docent explained that at fifty-nine degrees or below, the coastal moisture becomes so heavy on their wings they cannot fly.

Sometimes I feel like the monarch, as if I'm held down by the weight of my situation. A year later, having a husband with cancer still elicits powerful feelings of grief.

When your husband has cancer, there are many things to grieve. I am learning about and processing the losses we face. We are all searching for answers to difficult questions. All of us are touched by cancer, which brings us to the place of experiencing this journey. Some of us are just beginning while others are way ahead. Cancer changes life forever. But wherever you find yourself, you will have questions: *How do I live with a husband with cancer? How do I live with cancer? How do I say good-bye? How do I say good-bye to parts of my body? How do I say good-bye to parts of my spouse's body that don't work anymore? How do I say good-bye to my husband who once was joyful and is now depressed?* For some: *How do I save this relationship that I am losing?* There are so many losses during the cancer experience.

I have grieved periodically over the year, but not to this extent. It is normal for grief to come and go, but for now it has come again. Elizabeth Kübler-Ross and David Kessler wrote about the five phases of grief, which you may know: denial, anger, bargaining, depression, and acceptance.[8] When I was an RN on an oncology unit years ago, it was thought that you progressed from one stage to the next. In my practice, I have not seen that. Some stay in a phase, some never get to a phase at all, some go back and experience it all again. I experience the phases and revisit time and again. My grief is intensified when other life losses, ones unrelated to cancer, hit me. Losses such as a child leaving home.

I am recognizing and feeling pain from the loss. Only last month we went back to UCSF because penile injections were not working. In a funny way, I was relieved because I did not like injections. Sometimes they worked and sometimes they didn't. However, soon I realized it was one more attempt to get our love life back, and our best attempt failed again. Moving forward, we filled a new prescription of ED medication, but we discovered it was less effective than the medication Rick was already taking.

We attempted to use the new prescription during our Valentine's celebration, expecting better results. It didn't work at all. This failure caused Rick to retreat into himself.

---

8 http://grief.com/the-five-stages-of-grief/ accessed 8/6/2012.

I mourned my husband, our close body contact, and us. We had gotten somewhat closer, enjoying each other, and then bam, he was gone again. We were desperately hoping for the right conditions and then experienced so much disappointment. After 365 days of penile rehab, where did it get us? So I am in the anger phase. As life goes, I'm deeply entrenched. Last week, my best friend died. She had been struggling with cancer for a whole year. Today I had a question, and I thought, *I'll just ask my friend.* Then in that second of disbelief and reality, I felt the burst of shock and pain that she is gone. The anger seems to be building with each new development of life. A couple of days after our friend died, our son had an interview for a post-doctorate position in Vermont. We had hoped he would be moving back to California. While we were happy for him for this amazing opportunity, once again another layer of grieving had been added. More and more anger is surfacing within me.

Sharing deeply and personally opens the possibility for us to become aware of our thoughts and feelings. Grieving is nothing to be ashamed of. Learning where you are, being gracious to yourself, and finding the good in this will help get through this pain. I hope that if you find yourself, like me, starting, returning to, or finishing this grief work that you hold yourself closely with a gracious heart.

A line in the Serenity Prayer says it this way: "God, grant me serenity to accept the things I cannot change ... Accept hardships as a pathway to peace. Taking as Jesus did, this sinful world as it is, not as I would have it ... Amen."[9]

When I focus on the phrase, "Accept hardship as a pathway to peace," my first thought is, *No way. I do not find peace in the hardness of life. If anything, I become more anxious, afraid, and currently angry.* But then at a closer glance, it is not the hardness that brings peace but rather the acceptance of it. When I get to "It is what it

---

9   http://www.goodreads.com/author/quotes/31146.Reinhold_ Niebuhr, accessed 10/18/12.

is," and "I don't have to like it," I can become more at peace, gracious, and accepting.

Recently I received a call from a close relative that her husband had just been diagnosed with Glioblastoma, the worst grade of brain tumor. Hearing this news reminded me of the questions that popped into my mind when Rick was diagnosed with prostate cancer—such as: *What does that mean for the longevity of my spouse? Is this a death sentence? What do I tell my children? What does all this medical language mean? What are the parameters of this diagnosis? What is the prognosis? Is this hopeless?*

Each of us has unique questions regarding the unwelcome change in our circumstances. Each of these questions elicit all kinds of feelings. Some of these thoughts lead to a deepening of the grieving process, and others lead to resolving it. When my relative received the awful news, she thought her situation was hopeless. She assumed her husband would die very soon.

God graciously placed in my heart to share with her the thought that I know three people with this same diagnosis. All of them are still living ten years after their surgeries. Pausing, she said that gave her hope where she didn't have any before. I began calling my friends who have a deep faith and asked them to pray. These thoughts gave me great strength when inside I had been afraid. The cancer was twisted around his brain with tentacles, which meant it may not have been possible to remove all the cancer. Following surgery, we received the amazing news that total gross resection had been obtained, meaning all the cancer was removed.

While this was going on, one of my friends was praying for him and his family. In prayer, the friend said: "May the Lord do amazingly more than we could ever think or imagine—all for His glory!" God answered that powerful prayer.

This was *much* more than we could have imagined!

God, you are amazing. Listen to your thoughts. Listen to yourself, your prayers, because thoughts do affect the grieving process in a positive or negative way. Will your hardship keep you in the hardship or be that pathway to peace?

Even though the question of, "Will my spouse live?" was answered for us with a yes, I find myself periodically quite afraid. How quickly life turns on a dime. Even though God showed us great mercy in telling us through his surgeon that he feels Rick is cured from cancer and that our family member was told that they got it all, I feel so vulnerable. Life is so vulnerable. The words from Psalm 121:1 come to my mind: "I look to the hills where my help comes from."

The Bible verse I read today was Joshua 1:9: "Have I not commanded you? Be strong and of good courage; do not be afraid, nor be dismayed, for the LORD your God is with you wherever you go." As I read this verse through the filter of God, who holds me in His arms lovingly, I am calmed. When I read this verse with the knowledge that these are the arms and hands that cause a butterfly to take flight and galaxies to exist, I am encouraged. It is for these situations that God says be strong and not to be discouraged, for He knows we will be weak from time to time, and He knows we will be discouraged in this life, for this is not our permanent home.

If well-meaning friends or fellow Christians tell you not to be angry or afraid, remember that our Lord encourages us to be strong and encouraged because He knows we will feel a lot of things, grief included. Jesus wept. If our Lord wept, we surely can do so as well. Jesus accepts us where we are beginning, as He understands us completely.

Yesterday would have been the birthday of my friend who passed away. Rick and I found ourselves heading to the restaurant where we'd shared a meal with her once a month. Longingly, we wished we could be bringing her a gift as she had for us many times. We missed her laugh, her mischievous glances, and her deep love for us. We remembered the many times we shared our lives and felt her love once more. Moments of comfort are what I seek and pray for now to get through this grieving. Remembering was a moment of comfort.

Today Rick has success with his ED medication. This too was a moment of comfort through the darker feelings of loss because we once again achieved the close body comfort that creates a feeling of safety during a time I feel unsafe. God is faithful to provide moments of comfort as I look for them each new day.

Typically over the years I head to the garden when I am grieving. Some work harder to forget the pain, and some exercise profusely. Anything physical to reduce the frustrations of life is helpful. When I take a shovel and pound the ground to loosen it, I feel a physical lightening; it's my place to release anger. When I was a child, I grew up in a Christian community that taught all you need is faith, which discouraged expression of feelings. I was taught to put a lid on my feelings, which only served to intensify them. So today, I serve a Lord who can hear every expression of my anger as I work the land, and I release them into His loving hands where He can redeem them and restore me. It is there where I can have a voice about the current atrocities thrown at me, where I can cry and ask why, where I can say, "I'm angry that you've taken people and life's pleasures away from me."

When I spend the day pounding the earth, preparing the land, and then planting in my garden, I feel it releases me. As I dig the holes, I see myself letting go of some of the intense angst and frustration. I allow myself to say whatever it is I need to say, even what may seem inappropriate, and let it go into the deep earth. I fill the hole with gorgeous, blooming, full-of-life flowers.

I am deeply reminded that our loving Father promises good will come out of hardship. I think of my loved ones I miss because they moved, died, or changed, and I wonder what I can do to honor them in memory in the garden. For my ninety-five-year-old aunt, I hung a bird feeder. Every time I look at it, I remember her saying her calming words, "Can't get too riled up about these things." She lives on. As for Rick's prostate cancer, I'm placing a new loveseat in my garden in his honor and my commitment to enjoy each other and remember what we have endured together and what joys we still have to come.

Charles Spurgeon speaks of the deepest commitment we have from God to assist us along the way through the adversities of prostate cancer. I like to reflect on one of my favorite verses, Exodus 33:14, "My presence will go with you, and I will give you rest." Spurgeon uses the symbolism of two golden rings given to us from God. He sees two rings, one being His mighty powerful authoritative presence always with us, and the second God's promise to provide us with rest along these arduous journeys. This symbolism paints a clear picture of God placing these golden rings on our fingers. This is not just a marriage, as many see marriage today as easily broken, but a covenant that He would do anything, even die for us, because He is so captivated with us as His children. At times when I lose my way by doubting His love or begin to lose my sense of God's grace and presence, I look to these golden rings on my finger as a reminder of God's love and Rick's love.

As we find ourselves searching and grieving, I hope and pray we will see our hardship as a pathway to approaching calm. I surely am an example of the fallen, grounded butterfly in Pacific Grove, usually preferring to run away from grief and pain and not dealing with it. Grounded from the weight of the dire diagnosis and effects of treatment, I could not take flight. The heaviness of grieving keeps me down at times, but with help of others and God, I am confronting it. Like the monarch butterfly, I hope we all fly again after being temporarily grounded.

Questions/Thoughts
to Consider

1. Has the weight of a diagnosis of prostate cancer brought about a downcast spirit in either of you? If so, in what way?

2. Share the ways you've dealt with loss in the past.

3. Are there thoughts, feelings, or actions you take in order to avoid grieving?

4. Make a list of things that have changed since surgery. Which are unpleasant changes? Look at the losses you'll need to grieve.

5. Have your partner make a list. Share your lists with each other, then share your grief together. Since grieving is not a one-time event, agree to share your grief, as you become aware of it.

6. What do you know about God that brings you strength and comfort during this time?

Chapter 41

Let's Not Get Physical

As wives, we all have a lot of questions and concerns about our husbands' condition after surgery. So much is unknown and unfamiliar. Your husband may say these thoughts out loud or keep them to himself, but he will wonder if he is now unattractive, repulsive, or less of a man. A friend of mine, whose husband had prostate cancer, offered wise advice. She said the most important things you can offer your husband are companionship, understanding, encouragement, and ongoing love. Her words and prayers sustained me.

As I share the extent of my experience with Rick and my responses to recovering sexually, hopefully my experiences will provide you with comfort, affirmation, and support. You are not alone. There are some choices to make that will assist you through this difficult adversity. As wives, we can assist our husbands through recovery.

The night before Rick's prostatectomy, I questioned him once again: "Are you sure you want to do this?" It was important to know Rick was willing to risk losing urinary control and his erectile functioning in order to treat his cancer. I needed to be reassured that getting rid of the cancer was still his top priority.

At that time, he strongly declared, "I can't live with the fear of cancer destroying my life. I want the surgery."

I understood that completely as we both are imaginative worriers, and we would have been destroyed by worry. Yet I knew Rick lived his entire married life with me as a virile man, and it was his utmost priority. I trembled inside as we vowed that whatever the outcome, we would be there for each other.

Two days after surgery, we left UCSF. The rain was pouring so hard you couldn't see. As we approached the Bay Bridge, an expansive rainbow straddled it on either side, as if to say, "I, the Lord your God, am with you. It's going to be okay." It was obvious to me my husband was in great distress. Every bump and turn caused severe pain, and we still had a long drive home. Reality was sinking in.

When it was time for bed, we discovered that lying flat intensified his bladder spasms. We decided Rick would be more comfortable sleeping in a recliner next to our bed. Even though he was close, I sensed the emptiness and coldness because Rick's body was not snuggled next to mine. I cried deeply and silently that night.

The next two weeks went fairly well as Rick adjusted to having a catheter. His pain was well controlled. His healing from robotic surgery was amazingly quick. On the first morning home, Rick was ready for walks and to get out of the house. He was counting the days until his catheter would be removed. I remember quipping, "Be careful what you wish for."

Ostensibly, one could argue that Rick was doing great and that our family was falling back into routines, and outwardly that would look to be true. We did not yet have the pathology report, but familiar routines, such as teaching our daughter, Kate, and driving her to testing for home schooling kept me busy. Our youngest son had just moved into his own place in preparation for his upcoming wedding in two months. In two months, after sixteen years of being my children's teacher, all our children would move on to college. One would think I had a lot to look forward to.

Delving deeper into our hearts, we experienced the pain that came with mounting changes. The biggest was yet to come. On the first day his catheter was removed, it appeared Rick had some urinary control. He was able to start a urine flow on his first day, which raised our hopes. This control lasted a few hours. By nighttime he was fatigued. There was a stream of urine pouring out of my husband's penis. He had no control. As his wife, I felt deeply sad, like a major part of us had just been lost. I shared my grieving in my prayers and prayed for urological healing. The following verse came to mind: "Those who sow in tears shall reap in joy" (Psalm 126:5).

I wasn't devastated or disgusted, just sad—very sad. Subjectively, I was doing awful, yet objectively, I knew the God who created this Earth was still in control. Seeing urine didn't bother me as a nurse. A new care plan kicked in, and we had to do what needed to be done. I knew about incontinence, but I had never seen my husband incontinent. Rick began wearing diapers. As Rick lay next to me that night, I tried not to think about my husband in diapers. I realized nothing would be the same again.

A few days later, when Rick received his pathology report, we were relieved. We began sharing the great news with all who prayed for us. Our church gave us the opportunity to share our experiences at a worship service. We were grateful God answered our prayers to heal Rick from cancer. This was a joyful celebration as we saw God's hand in this, and it was great to feel joy instead of fear and sadness.

Quickly, like living in two worlds side by side, the other reality surfaced. Rick began to recover quickly from surgery. At the same time he experienced painful debilitating emotions. This began when he found that trips away from home resulted in his arriving back home with urine-soaked pants. Often he ran to the bathroom as he felt a frequent urgency to use a bathroom. At this point Rick had no idea how often to change his diapers, how to stay dry, how many Kegels he should do, and what he could do to prevent his frequent and painful bladder spasms.

More and more I found Rick sitting in his recliner with computer in hand attempting to keep up with work. His desire to leave home or engage with the world was rapidly diminishing. Our conversation changed from our goal of being cancer free to being urine free. Now Rick would say, "If only I wasn't incontinent, I could live with ED." Would we ever see urine control? His urologist had warned him based on his urological history there was a possibility he'd never regain urinary control. Hearing this warning was frightening. Watching Rick live out that reality was a disaster. Not only was this happening to Rick, it was happening to us. This experience was the beginning of the tearing down of our relationship.

Attention to the minute details of urinary control began to be the majority of our conversations. What was the progression of recovery from incontinence? We researched together the many top medical institutions across the nation to determine what should be happening. Watching earnestly, we waited for nighttime dryness, early morning dry times, and then our most coveted dry in the evening. Intense vigilance over systemic problems and treatments, monitoring medications and the side-effects, and evaluating effectiveness of treatments was what we talked about. Even though we were communicating often, the effects of the cancer began to take their toll. I prayed for wisdom, for God to ease Rick's suffering, and for our Lord's grace to meet up with the mountain of cancer-related problems.

I loved Zephaniah 3:17: "The LORD your God in your midst, the mighty One, will save; He will rejoice over you with gladness, He will quiet you with His love, He will rejoice over you with singing."

My insides needed quieting. I was powerless, and I knew my Savior redeems not only in salvation but in every situation in life. All the while we were living with urological issues, the research showed the necessity of bringing oxygenated blood supply to the penis. I took it upon myself to begin this process, which is called penile rehabilitation (PR). The first few attempts were received reluctantly as Rick's awareness of what he lost was evident. It was not left unnoticed to me, however, that in spite of my womanly wiles, Rick could not become erect. I felt sadness and discouraged because at some level I knew this could destroy us. Intently, I kept focusing on the progress and the consequences of loss of function if we gave up on PR.

After a few days of Rick's failure to experience an erection, he wanted nothing more to do with PR until he had some urinary control. Frustrated, we discussed the need to keep going yet we knew and accepted that he needed a break. We were able to share together physically doing things differently. We shared some enjoyable sexual experiences, but both of us recognized the post-surgical changes. It was painful to lose Rick's responsiveness, attention, and interest in sex.

It hurt to have a husband who lost his interest in pursuing me. Deep grieving began. I knew I could grieve to my God and expect great comfort from Him. I was confident that He would make good out of a horrible time, yet I cried, releasing the frustrations into His loving arms. But with all the bad, this time I knew God loved me all the time, good or bad.

Increasingly, Rick took to his chair and computer and remained there most of the day except for our daily walks. The discouragement he felt being in diapers was profound. The lack of control of his body led to retreating from people. He did not visit with friends who asked to come over. Many days I felt shut out. On rare occasions, we shared our fears of things never getting better. When we saw some progress with Rick's urinary control, we shared our joy.

Our first time out together other than doctor's appointments was to walk to a floral nursery. Learning the hard way, we had to leave as soon as we got there because there wasn't a bathroom and Rick didn't want to urinate in his diaper. We were attempting to do something other than deal with cancer. We were attempting to do something that I liked to do.

I needed a break from the mounting stresses and needed to live life. About a month out, we knew we needed to add fun to our lives, so we went to a Steven Curtis Chapman concert. We loved being out. Uncertainty of where bathrooms were and fears of leaking though diapers were present, but I appreciated Rick's effort to take me out under such conditions. Painstakingly slow around the sixth-week post-op, we realized the return of urinary control in the early mornings. It would be present and then gone for a couple of days but then return to being dry every morning. By the tenth week, we noticed a pattern. Rick could stay dry until late afternoon. By nighttime he was severely leaking again. During this phase, we felt we could only deal with the urine control progress.

Even though this time was wrought with disappointment every day, I looked for God's way of comforting me, showing me He was around, and bringing strength to me. I saw these each and every day. Sometimes it was as simple as seeing a butterfly, which reassured me of His providential care for His creation. It was though I was kissed by God.

Some researchers documented progress from ED up until the eighth week. We did see little glimpses of improvement, and it brought hope. Yet at that benchmark all progress stopped, if not regressed. We became discouraged. We kept up with PR, although it was becoming a chore rather than an activity that gave either of us any pleasure. All semblance of romance was gone. It was what had to be done. Many times Rick would talk about issues at work or what had to be done for the day during the rehab. The *us* that we once knew was going away.

We decided at the ten-week checkup at UCSF we would discuss further treatment for ED. Would there be help? Would Rick recover from dysfunction? We felt increasingly agitated because we both wanted Rick's manliness back. At the ten-week follow-up appointment, we emerged very happy. Our surgeon had just told us he dared to say Rick was healed. Not only that, but three days before the appointment, the urgency incontinence had stopped, as if a faucet was just shut off. We were so happy. Rick also requested a pump for penile rehab. The staff recommended penile injections for ED, but Rick said he would never do that. We celebrated the news of Rick being cured from cancer by having dinner overlooking the San Francisco Bay. We were overjoyed and hopeful that like the progress with incontinence, we would see progress with ED. The staff was confident Rick's sexual function would return to its level prior to surgery. We thanked the Lord, the Great Physician, for Rick's healing. Both of us are grateful for the news that Rick was healed from cancer!

Only a week later, our thirty-first anniversary was here. Unconsciously, the tension mounted. Consciously, we made plans to go away alone. I think I still hoped going away would awaken those sleeping nerve bundles. Rick seemed distracted with work. I wondered whether Rick's failure to obtain a useable erection with the pump was affecting our relationship in a negative way. I suspected we were heading for disaster. Let's get physical—or were we telling each other, "Let's not get physical"?

All those expectations and two tired, angry partners coming to grips with reality plowed us over. We were two silent people attempting to love one another under such conditions, recognizing we were drifting far apart. Our closeness was gone. I remember crying out, "Please come back to me." Looking back, I can see he was extremely depressed and had left me long ago.

Feeling totally ignored, I asked Rick if he wanted to stay married to me. I was ready to stop trying to keep our relationship together because I couldn't take being rejected anymore. As in most of my arguments with Rick, I wish I knew how to bring these truths with more grace and less pain. He had enough going on, and so did I. We were both in deep pain. On our way home, at least we came to that conclusion. We stopped for an ice cream sundae. This brief time of fun helped us come back together again.

When we returned home, we were confronted with another loss. When Chris returned from his honeymoon he found a new job. This meant he'd no longer be working at our restaurants. We were very happy for Chris and his wife, Bre. We were also reminded that we were in a completely different phase in our marriage that neither of us wanted to be in. Chris was in a season of new beginnings, and we were in a season of new and frequent losses. Now it would be on Rick's shoulders to run both stores without Chris's help. This meant Rick would have a lot more to do. We tried to make the best of it. We attempted to be attentive to one another, but being attentive also reminded us of what we no longer had available to us.

The summer seems a blur. I remember going swimming only a couple of times because we were just too tired and it was already July. We both told each other we needed fun in our lives. Swimming was relaxing and brought us physically together, which felt great. Reflecting, it felt like I was three months behind. I hadn't even planted a flower yet.

We continued with penile rehab. Rick began using ED medication and the pump at the same time. We were both disappointed that Rick remained unable to achieve a useable erection. We found other ways to please one another, and that felt great. We also continued to feel great loss about what had been. Discouraged with the lack of progress and the fear of developing a venous leak, Rick was ready to try penile injections. We once again wanted to feel hopeful yet had been burned by the pump and the failure to achieve an erection with medication. We were cautious and didn't want to get our hopes up that injecting would be successful.

Six months after surgery, we went back to UCSF to see the ED specialist so Rick could learn how to perform penile injections. He injected himself on the first visit. The nurse practitioner was certain that once we found the correct dosage, Rick would have success injecting. He was given a prescription for Bi-mix. Believing we would have success, we left UCSF very encouraged.

The first injection took a long time to take effect. Our brains were working on overload, taking over our natural physical desires, but the injection worked. We found ourselves creating a number system (from one to ten) the hardness of Rick's erections. An eight was very rigid and useable while a three had some level of hardness but was not useable.

For the first time in three months, we experienced making love again. It wasn't romantic. It was full of techniques and the distraction of the injection, but we were delighted we could experience physical oneness again.

After three months of successfully injecting, Rick stopped experiencing useable erections. Pained with not only the discomfort of the injection but emotional discomfort of living with the thought of being less than a man, once again I felt Rick's rejection of sex, which included me. By now, I knew he was struggling with the failure of injections, but I felt as though it was my personal failure. I felt rejected. After all, there was nothing I could do to arouse him. Rick became pretty passive about this whole thing. I was frustrated. I had lost my leader.

During Rick's recovery, I had a hysterectomy. During my recovery, I was one of the fortunate (or unfortunate in this case) women to become more interested in making love. I approached my husband encouragingly after the doctor gave me the all clear. Even though I was a bit frightened to do it after surgery, I was ready. I shared the good news that I was cleared medically. I did not receive excitement but defensiveness. I felt discouraged. I was driven to keep Rick interested in penile rehab even though he was discouraged and seemed ready to give up. My own interest waxed and waned too, but I knew the importance of the rehab to maintain penile function. I desired our closeness in lovemaking, and I knew the importance of sex to Rick even though it hurt him greatly in the moment.

After five months of injections, it was clear Rick was no longer responding to them. Physical stimulation plus the use of ED medication was working better than injections, but Rick could not attain a useable erection. So we went back to the UCSF ED specialist. She could not understand why the injections had suddenly failed. She had Rick inject a different medication. As Rick injected the Tri-mix, she said there was nothing wrong with his technique. Rick's level of hardness with Tri-mix was between two and three. It was not a useable erection. She said it was possible a larger dose of tri-mix would work. Rick was in so much pain from the injection, there was no way he would inject another dose of Tri-mix. While we both were disappointed injections stopped working, there was also some relief. We were offered a different ED medication that stayed in the body for a longer period of time.

Now eleven months post-surgery, we left that office kind of numb and with a greatly diminished expectation of success. Regardless of the outcome of that day, we were determined to enjoy the rest of the day. Our daughter, Kate, had come with us. She and I had a wonderful time shopping. Rick kept to himself because he was in too much pain.

On the drive home we decided we'd spend a few days away for Valentine's Day. We both believed we'd have a better time than we did six months earlier for our anniversary. That's when we'd tried the pump with no success. Our Valentine's celebration brought us mentally, emotionally, and spiritually closer. Notice I didn't say physically. We tried the new medication, which was better because it seemed to put Rick in the mood, which had been vacant up until now. But Rick experienced severe back pain. Maybe it wasn't such a good idea to try something new when we were getting away to enjoy time together and have fun.

Three months later we've been hobbling along. Rick would occasionally have a useable erection, but there were many failed attempts. Rick stopped taking the medication that gave him backaches and went back to the medication he took after the penile injections failed. We continued to see some progress with useable erections, which we both enjoyed very much.

After his yearly checkup, Rick had to add another blood pressure medication to his list of medications. One possible side-effect was erectile dysfunction. I thought we'd both need a new arsenal of motivation to keep going. After a couple of weeks on the new medication, Rick was still able to obtain a useable erection. I rejoiced! After sixteen months, I wish I could say Rick has fully recovered both urinary control and his erectile function, but that is not the case. For some of the men reading this, you may experience a full return of both urinary and erectile functions early on. If this doesn't happen, I hope you women won't give up on your husband or your relationship. Each case is as individual as fingerprints. There is no doubt we can learn from one another, but know your experience is your own.

When I read and reread what Rick and I have endured, I see the depth of isolation prostate cancer brings the patient and the spouse. I did not feel comfortable sharing the intricacies of my pain. Yet I was able to support and be supported by a couple going through the same diagnosis with different functioning abilities. I'm grateful to them!

If you are given an opportunity to share with others, it brings strength. Talking with your partner also clarifies misunderstandings and brings an emotional connection to prepare for sexual activity. There is a tendency to protect our partners to not harm them and keep things to ourselves. This only brings more grief and separation and isolation. When you feel isolated, sad, and angry or whatever painful emotions share them with each other. Who knows? Your partner may also feel some of these things.

We, as ladies, share many experiences of this life with prostate cancer. There are others who know this life too. You are not alone. It does get better. Ask for what you need. Rely on our heavenly Father to guide and offer a shoulder to carry you through.

Questions/Thoughts to Consider

1. Notice your thoughts and responses to your partner if he withdraws from you.

2. How will you deal with your hurt, and sense of rejection?

3. Can you discuss your feelings without the presence of anger or defensiveness?   If not, what does that tell you?

4. Are one or both of you avoiding sex? If so, how is that choice affecting your relationship?

5. Some women experience a sense of relief when their husband loses his desire and/or his ability for sex. Do you? If so, why? If not, what can you to do maintain your physical relationship?

6. It is possible to become so desperate for emotional and/or physical attention, one or both of you could experience the temptation to have an emotional and/or physical affair. If you experience this temptation, will you give in or fight for your marriage?

Chapter 42

Final Thoughts

As I realize the depth of adversity during recovery from prostate surgery for Rick and me, I now see how much I have tried to lighten the load and remain upbeat by looking for the good in the suffering. I have been blessed by seeking, and I have seen God's mercies every day. Yet it may have also been my attempt to avoid staying in the season of suffering. I wanted to hurry up and live life again. Many times Rick was not there with me. Many times I felt alone. Yet I pressed forward, perhaps too quickly. Skipping ahead may have caused me to lose what God has in mind for me to see. One such example occurred recently. Speaking to God daily through prayer brought me to the end of myself. I realized that when I ended, there was nothing left—no more fear, no more sadness. There I find that this battle is the Lord's. It is His sword and shield that fights this battle. There is peace here. There is calm here. He is omnipotent. I am insecure and overwhelmed, but with Him I am strengthened to go on in a more peaceful place, awaiting His grace to meet up with the next struggle. Nothing is too hard for Him.

In the "new normal" ahead of me, I am letting go of wishing things were back to the old normal. I'm grieving too many changes, too many losses, too much lack of familiarity, and too many unknowns. With Jesus' mercy I go ahead, realizing I don't have to like it. I certainly don't like the pain and suffering, but I do like the realization that God is working this out for my good. Like blown glass in the fire, I am being molded into His image. Like molecules of carbon form a diamond, I am being heated and pressurized to form a gem—a gem that He cherishes.

In this process of illness and recovery, I see myself becoming more Christ-like, more trusting and sanctified. I'm becoming more the person our Lord desires me to be, knowing I am loved in good and bad times. Never abandoning, our Lord stays at our side, speaking softly to our tender hearts. He knows what we need from His many promises and new mercies for each day.

This has been a difficult journey. I wish I could end this chapter telling you this ED problem is resolved. Instead, I'll tell you nineteen months after surgery, it's still a struggle. In the coming year we hope for continued improvement. I hope your journey may be shorter, with a quicker recovery. If it is not, I certainly wish you the best and hope that by sharing our struggles, we provided you with insight and encouragement to cope with the post-surgical issues that will affect your relationship.

Bibliography

American Cancer Society, "What Are the Key Statistics about Prostate Cancer?" Last modified February 27, 2012. Accessed April 4, 2012. http://www.cancer.org/Cancer/ProstateCancer/DetailedGuide/prostate-cancer-key-statistics.

Chodak, Gerald. *Winning the Battle Against Prostate Cancer: Get the Treatment That Is Right For You* (New York: Demos Medical Publishing, 2011).

Geisler, Norman L. *Christian Apologetics* (Grand Rapids, MI: Baker Books, 2006).

Gilbertson, Jim. PC Study Bible for Windows, NKJV, version 3.2F. Seattle: Biblesoft, 1988. Computer software.

Gottman, John M. and Julie Schwartz Gottman. *Ten Lessons to Transform Your Marriage* (New York: Three Rivers Press, 2006).

Gottman, John M. and Nan Silver. *The Seven Principles for Making Your Marriage Work* (New York: Random House, 1999), 115.

———. "Marriage Styles: The Good, the Bad, and the Volatile," *Why Marriages Succeed or Fail.* (New York: Simon & Schuster, 1994), 57.

Klein, Allen. *The Healing Power of Humor* (New York: Penguin, 1989), 49.

Kübler-Ross, Elisabeth and David Kessler. "The Five Stages of Grief." http://grief.com/the-five-stages-of-grief. Accessed August 6, 2012.

McDonald, Gordon. "Storms Happen." *In the Life God Blesses 19.* (Nashville, TN: Thomas Nelson, 1994).

McDowell, Josh. *More Than a Carpenter*, First Edition (Wheaton, IL: Tyndale House Publishers, 1987).

Mulhall, John P. YouTube video, "Penile Rehabilitation after Cancer Treatment," accessed April 10, 2011, http://www.youtube.com/watch?v=ie8NkOu2VNA.

————. *Saving Your Sex Life: A Guide for Men With Prostate Cancer* (Bethesda, MD: C-I-ACT Publishing, 2010).

Mullins, Nicole C. "My Redeemer Lives," accessed April 10, 2011, http://www.lyricsty.com/nicole-c-mullins-my-redeemer-lives-lyrics.html.

Newsboys. "Blessed Be Your Name," YouTube video, accessed February 2, 2011, http://www.youtube.com/watch?v=DLycgKxlgc0wsboys.

Niebuhr, Reinhold. "Serenity Prayer," Accessed October 18, 2012,

www.goodreads.com/author/quotes/31146.

Parker-Pope, Tara. "Regrets after Prostate Surgery," August 27, 2008. Accessed February 18, 2012, http://well.blogs.nytimes.com/2008/08/27/regrets-after-prostate-surgery/.

Rosberg, Gary. *Do-It-Yourself Relationship Mender* (Colorado Springs, CO: Focus on the Family, 1992).

Smalley, Greg, Robert S. Paul, and Donna K. Wallace. *The DNA of Relationships for Couples.* (Carol Stream, IL: Tyndale Publishing Inc., 2006).

Smith, Michael, W., Israel Huston. "Help Is on the Way," YouTube Video, accessed February 7, 2011, http://www.ehow.com/how_12107048_cite-youtube.html

Spurgeon, Charles H. and Roy H. Clark, Ed. *Beside Still Waters* (Nashville, TN: Thomas Nelson, 1998).

Story, Laura. "Blessings," Story behind the Song, accessed March 2011. http://www.youtube.com/results?search_query=the+blessing+laura+story+behind+the+song&oq=the+blessing+laura+story+behind+the+song&gs_l=youtube.3 ... 4088.9732.0.9864.16.15.0.0.0.0.182.1475.8j6.14.0 ... 0.0 ... 1ac.DS6J-gVJRWk.

———. K-Love, Laura Story, "Blessings" Live, YouTube Video, March 2, 2012 http://www.youtube.com/watch?v=1CSVqHcdhXQ.

Strobel, Lee. *The Case for Faith* (Grand Rapids, MI: Zondervan, 2000).

Thomas, Gary. *Sacred Marriage: What If God Designed Marriage to Make Us Holy More than to Make Us Happy?* (Grand Rapids, MI: Zondervan, 2000).

_____. *Pure Pleasure.* (Grand Rapids, MI: Zondervan, 2009).

Walsh, Patrick C. and Janet F. Worthington. *Guide to Surviving Prostate Cancer*, Second Edition (New York: Wellness Central, 2007).

Online Resources for Information and Support

MD Junction Prostate Cancer Support Group:
http://www.mdjunction.com/prostate-cancer

The New Prostate Cancer Info Link—Prostate Cancer
Support Group: http://prostatecancerinfolink.net/
questions/ask-arnon/

Prostate Cancer Support Association:
http://www.prostatecancersupport.info/

A Prostate Cancer Support Forum:
http://www.healingwell.com/community/default.aspx

A support group for men with erectile dysfunction: http://
www.franktalk.org/Enter.php?redirect=/index.php

Prostate Cancer Foundation will help to find a prostate
cancer support group near you:
http://www.pcf.org/site/c.leJRIROrEpH/b.5699537/k.BEF4/Home.
htm

A prostate cancer support group for wives and partners:
http://www.hisprostatecancer.com/prostate-cancer-support-
groups.html

Women against Prostate Cancer:
http://www.womenagainstprostatecancer.org/

About the Authors

Rick Redner received in master's degree in social work at Michigan State University and worked as a medical social worker for two years. For the last thirty years he's been self-employed as the owner and operator of two sandwich shops in Modesto, California. He was diagnosed with prostate cancer at age fifty-eight.

To contact Rick for any reason, including speaking engagements, e-mail whereisyourprostate@gmail.com.

Brenda Redner received her RN/BSN at Michigan State University. She's worked as an oncology nurse, psychiatric nurse, and teacher. She left nursing in order to home school all four of their children. She was fifty-six when her husband was diagnosed with prostate cancer.

To contact Brenda for any reason, including speaking engagements, e-mail whereishisprostate@gmail.com.

Please visit us frequently at www.whereisyourprostate.com.